MW01274408

101 Reasons To Have Sex
&
Just As Many Reasons Not To

Dianne Wyntjes

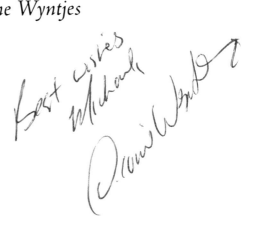

Bloomington, IN   authorHOUSE®   Milton Keynes, UK

AuthorHouse™
1663 Liberty Drive, Suite 200
Bloomington, IN 47403
www.authorhouse.com
Phone: 1-800-839-8640

AuthorHouse™ UK Ltd.
500 Avebury Boulevard
Central Milton Keynes, MK9 2BE
www.authorhouse.co.uk
Phone: 08001974150

This book is a non-clinical approach to the twists and turns of intimate relations. It is not to be construed as psychological or medical advice. Seek professional assistance from your doctor.

First published by AuthorHouse   11/21/2006

ISBN: 978-1-4259-6996-7 (sc)
ISBN: 978-1-4259-6995-0 (hc)

Editor: Roxane Christ, Vancouver, British Columbia, Canada

Printed in the United States of America
Bloomington, Indiana

This book is printed on acid-free paper.

To

Allan, my love, who inspires me.

And to you, the reader.

I've come to know many reasons to have sex and many reasons not to. I've learned many lessons in my search for a healthy and blessed relationship. I share them with you.

Enjoy your journey.

Contents

101 Reasons To Have Sex

& Just As Many Reasons Not To

101 Reasons To Have Sex

You're Such A Romantic And I Love You For It.

Some of us are born romantics at heart.
You know the kind of partner….
Loveable, huggy, kissy, touchy, feely, gift giving.
The one who remembers special occasions
and plans the outings;
The one who doesn't forget special occasions;
And is upset when you do.

For others, we must learn to become romantic.
Romance is:
A kiss when you leave in the morning, and one at night,
A message of love and good intentions,
A love letter.

Romance is doing things together
Such as taking a massage class,
And practicing on your partner.
Understanding, being supportive, giving a compliment.

A surprise gift of affection, loving actions,
Being loyal,
Holding hands, even when you don't want to….
It's the glow on their faces when something special exists between
two people.

Is romance waning in your relationship?
Is finding romance a chore?
You've got what you wanted,
The work is done.

What's the remedy?
Put the hours into your relationship,
Just like you put into your job,
There will be a payoff.

You were once a romantic.
It's time to re-create the romance,
Or the relationship will go stale.

I'm Bored, Sex Revives Me!

Sex is exciting in the beginning.
Over time, it changes.

In some cases, we may become complacent about our sexual activities.
We've lost the energy and passion.
You know—same old routine and familiarity.

The combination of communication, respect and sharing experiences creates
the essence of our relationships.

The ups and downs, the good times and bad times
engenders memories.
The resolve to make it work will take you to the
silver and golden years.

In today's day and age, we live in a disposable society.
We may feel disinterest and boredom.
We may stare at the ceiling and think, "Is this it?"
When something doesn't work,
We get rid of it and get something new.
That's not always the best action or reaction.

It's important to recognize that sex can be a vital ingredient
in your relationship.
Passionate and magical sex may not last forever,
Sometimes our relationships need resuscitation.

Relationships and good sex require work.
It takes interest and activity to make it happen.
Communication and commitment along with
being good friends leads you to being good lovers.

Make sex fun and keep the passion alive!
Good sex can revive and refresh you!
Smile if you're revitalized!

You Fulfill Many Needs In My Life.

Your partner can be a companion, a breadwinner,
a travel mate, a cook, a cleaner, a fixer, or a gardener,
Or whatever role you have them fill in your life.

Relationships require us to be many things
at many different times in our life.

But the most important roles are friends and lovers.
To know someone deeply,
To hear them,
To understand them,
To have them understand you,
To trust one another,
To cherish one another,
To inspire each other,
To choose them again,
If you had the chance.

You fulfill my needs.
You complement me.
You complete me.
We'll let our love grow.

It's My Birthday!

You should always get lucky on your birthday, if you want.
It's your special day.

If you wrestle with purchasing the perfect birthday present for your partner,
There are the dependable standbys:

For Men: She usually likes flowers and fragrance, chocolates, her favorite book, dinner and a movie, clothing, a new top-of-the line cell phone, a day at the spa, a gift certificate, travel, or simply, time together.

For Women: He usually likes a new electronic gadget or handyman tool, his favorite music, cologne, dinner and a movie, sports equipment, a gift certificate, your sexy underwear, travel, or simply, time together. Surprise him with flowers or a plant.

Enjoy the birthday in your birthday suit!
It's your day to initiate sex!
Wrap yourself in ribbons.
Most importantly, give the gift of yourself.

It's Our Anniversary.

Women are better at remembering special dates.
You know, the first month's anniversary when you met, the second month,
the seventh month, the first year,
And so it goes.

Men: take heed!
Women love to keep track of anniversaries,
and not just when you're married.

Recognize the special dates.
Try to remember them.
Put them in your day timer.
Have the neighborhood florist remind you.

At the same time, let your partner know that each day,
each month and each year together,
is important and precious.

If it's important to your partner, and it likely is,
Do something special to commemorate the day!

Yet, why do we need anniversaries
to celebrate our accomplishments?

Every day should be a celebration of our love for each other.

Happy anniversary, dear—today and everyday!

You're A Good Provider.

The comfort zone,
You know where you are in your relationship.
Familiarity and contentment,
Where you hang your coat and plunk your shoes.

To feel safe and to know things are looked after,
Where financial security is valued but emotional security is more important.

Good providers have a leg up in the romance department.
They experience fewer pressures so they can focus on other priorities, including focusing on their mate.
They want to get it right and please their partner.

Pleasures in your life,
And pleasures in your bedroom.

You're a fortunate person; count your blessings.
Be grateful for each other.

I Feel Your Vibes And You Feel Mine.

Intuition.
There's something between us.

Why is it that with some people we feel nothing?
With others, there's a connection,
A feeling,
Body language,
Chemistry,
Pheromones,
Signals,
There's a bond that becomes stronger,
You want to get to know the person better.

Unfinished business?

The vibes are definitely two-way.
The connection doesn't happen often,

When it does—go for it!

…And see what becomes of the spark.

You're Successful And That Turns Me On.

Successful people in life seem to be the ones who tackle
each day with gusto,
With a positive attitude.
They see the glass half-full, not half-empty.
They know that if today is a tough day,
Tomorrow can be better.
They have purpose.
They get to work on time.
They have goals and dreams.
They're reliable.
Trusting and considerate,
Patient and compassionate,
Giving positive reinforcement,
Appreciating each day,
And managing the twists and turns.

To be successful in your relationship,
Find someone with a similar moral code.
Find someone with the characteristics
that are endearing to you.
Then you will have a solid basis
For a good and healthy relationship.

Because You Are So Sexy....

What one person finds a turn-on,
Another may not.
That's a good thing.
We are all different.
Our attractions are unique to each of us.

Ever heard or commented, "They make a *strange couple!*"

If we all had the same attractions,
Life wouldn't be interesting.

Be sexy;
If you're a few pounds overweight—live large!
Be comfortable with your body.
Recognize your flaws and work for improvement.
Nobody's perfect.
If you're not happy—do something about it,
Stop having a negative or distorted image of your body,
Appreciate it and love it.
Get active,
Get a stylish haircut,
Or bald is beautiful.
You can be sexy at any age!

Accepting yourself is sexy.
Someone out there will be fascinated.
Be you.

We're Breaking Up And It's The Last Time....

We'll make love.

If you've ever ended a relationship,
You may understand the desire to have one last lover's romp;
One last time to share your emotion and passion.
Nostalgia and what might have been.

You both know it's the last time.
You're both mature enough to know
it will never happen again.
You're both moving on.

It's goodbye sex.

Then, all that remains is a memory.

I Feel Sorry For You!

You try so hard,
You look so desperate,
I don't want to turn you down.
I feel sorry for you!
It's sympathy.

Yes, sometimes just to make someone feel better,
Or good about themselves,
You sacrifice yourself,
A good deed,
One time only….
The mercy one.

Let's Do It Someplace Else, Besides The Bed.

Get out of the routine and your comfort zone.

In the kitchen,
In the shower,
On the couch,
Try it in every room in the house!

Then the back yard,
The bushes,
The beach,
The boat,
A strange hotel room,
… And for old times sake, the car!
Awaken the romance that has been asleep at the wheel.

You'll share laughter and memories.

The couple that plays together,
Stays together.

You're My Wish Come True.

I've been lonely so many times in my life,
Wishing and hoping for someone to be with me.

Simply because you wanted to,
You chose me
To share my time,
To make memories together.

I've wished upon the stars so many times,
And here you are,
Finally!

My family and friends told me to be patient,
To become the best I could be,
To wait for that special day,
When you'd walk into my life.

You're here and I feel so fortunate.
It was all worth it.

I can turn the page.
It's a new chapter in my life.
The best is yet to come.
We can wish upon the stars....
Together.

It's Valentine's Day.

A romantic day to celebrate our love!

A lover should pull out all the romantic moves on this day for the love of your life.
Be predictable with roses or flowers,
Chocolates,
Wine or champagne,
A gift of affection,
A ring, a heart shaped pendant, a bracelet that represents endless love,
Romantic love songs,
Close dancing.

Let yourself go,
Abandon yourself to the dizziness of emotion and love.

A good day to propose,
Or propose all over again.

February 14th is the definitive day of love and lust.
For red-hot lovers, everyday is a Love Day!
Every day is Valentine's Day!

Let's Have A Quickie!

The unexpected surprise when you're least expecting it.

Men, on average, ask for quickies more often.
Men, on average, enjoy quickies more than women.

Couples, on average, have more quickies when they're younger.

Women like the preparation, the teasing, the ambiance, and the foreplay.
Women like the cuddling and the intimate conversation—before and afterwards.

Men like the action and the sizzle.
Men like the release and satisfaction.
Sex is dessert for men!

But the memory of a quickie for both sexes
Will always bring a smile to your face when you think about it.

Try it—you'll like it!

It's Been A While; You've Been Away.

Being apart.

Traveling on business—again.
Distance can be a problem.
Not calling after 24 hours,
Are you that busy?
Or not interested in what's at home?
Take the time to call and share your day.
Put your partner at ease.

A phone connection and phone sex can be safe
and not messy,
But it's just not the same as face-to-face, cheek-to-cheek.

Home is not the same without your partner.
Their smell, their touch, their stuff lying around....

Enjoy the anticipation of seeing someone after a period of absence.
There's something about suppressed emotion and passion ready to spill.

Coming home to your own bed and companionship
Sure beats business travel,
And an empty hotel room.

Enjoy The Pleasures Of Life.

There are two kinds of pleasure:
Physical and
Emotional.

There are the physical things—good food, gifts and treasures, champagne, a fast car, a trip away, and decadence.
There are the pleasures of the flesh—your naked body, your scent, and the touch of your skin, how you taste....

But it's the emotional pleasures that reach me and leave me wanting more.
You're in my thoughts.
I feel so much emotion when we talk after sex.
We connect.

There's the lasting pleasure, the emotional pleasures
When you touch my heart with yours,
When we share our deepest thoughts,
Our hopes, fears and dreams.

It's the pleasures of the heart and mind,
That gives us precious memories,
And leads us into our future.

You Make Me Feel So Loved.

It's the special things you do.

The notes you tuck in my lunch with your silly drawings of
a heart, a happy face and special love thoughts,
The phone call mid day.
You don't want anything,
Just to let me know you're thinking about me.
The text message,
The special gifts you give me,
It's not my birthday, not our anniversary.
You thought of me and bought something, just for me.
You don't have to buy me bouquets of flowers,
A single stem will do.

So often in our relationship, you say "I love you."
At the unexpected times.
Say it often.
Show it often.
It's not just the words, it's the action.

Right before we go to sleep, you cuddle with me,
With a goodnight kiss.
Until morning, when you greet me with another kiss.
You wish me good things for the day ahead.

Sharing our life is an incredible journey.

You make me feel so loved.

I Feel I Can Trust You.

Sex and making love is a responsible activity.
A yearning that must be quenched.
It comes from lust, passion and love.

It comes from one of the above or all of the above.

In today's modern times, sex is serious.

Sex can have life altering consequences:
Bruised hearts,
Broken dreams,
Unwanted children,
And the most dreaded of all—sexually transmitted diseases.

Someone you can trust is a must.
Understanding that your partner needs his or her space is important and
you need to trust, without jealousy.
Being responsible is crucial:
Responsible to each other, and being responsible
Between the sheets.
Precautions are mandatory.
Plan your life.
Choose your partner carefully.

Use condoms for responsible sex.
Don't have sex, when in doubt.

I Need To Have Someone To Play With!

Playtime keeps you young.
Something left over from our childhood,
Being child like but not childish.

As an adult, you should still have playtime.
Find the time to play together,
Laugh together and have fun!

A romp in the sack on a lazy afternoon,
A roll in the grass in a farmer's field when you need a break from a long drive,
Be spontaneous,
Experiment,
Use your imagination!

Pull the covers over your head.
Giggle and tickle!

Sometimes the most intense emotional experiences
Aren't planned,
They just happen!

Isn't it fun to have someone to play with!
Be young at heart!
Show your spirit!

I Want To Get Lucky!

Luck is fortune bestowed by chance.
Or do we make our own luck by our attitude and reactions to life's twists and turns?

Anytime we have good sex and love combined,
We're fortunate.
Love is good.
Desire is powerful.
Sex is great.
When they're combined, it's magnificent!

Celebrate with your partner.
Enjoy each other.
Go for it and don't hold back!

If we're too cautious in love, we may be missing out on the happiness that's waiting for us.
There's never a guarantee that everything will be perfect.

Roll the dice on love and get lucky!

You're A Cougar On The Prowl And I Want Some Of That.

You know the kind:
Sexy and sassy,
All style,
Seductive,
A quiet self-confidence,
Naughty in a good way,
Flirty,
Witty,
Playful,
Makes eye contact,
A body that's well maintained,
A seasoned bombshell,
Maturity that's sexy,
Wisdom and experience,
No inhibitions in bed,
Knows her way around....

Purrs like a cat....
Meow!

You want some of that!

I Need To Sample The Goods Before I Choose.

Sex is like a box of chocolates.
Some can have just one and stop.
Others need to try a few before they find the one
They know is their flavor.

But remember when you sample,
You're dealing with heart and emotions.

While some may want just sex,
Others want the attachment, sentiments and the beginnings of a commitment.

Know yourself,
Know your destination,
Know what you want,
Think about the other person,
Before you open the box.

I Need To Sow My Wild Oats.

If that's what you need to do,
Make sure you do it before you're into a long-term relationship.
A one night stand is tempting, but is it worth it?

Some need to explore and experience different relationships to find the best
match for their own personality.

But don't leave a trail of broken hearts.

No one has an unbreakable heart.
Don't use and abuse,
Don't lead someone on,
Be sensitive to your lover's feelings.

Relationships are not like a wild meadow.
Rather, they're like a garden that needs attention.
We should be gardeners of our relationships,
Nurturing them.

Our love affairs are like a rosebush,
So beautiful and fragile,
Emerging into the light and full of new growth.
But watch the thorns; they can be painful.

Yes, wild oats can be sown,
But planting seeds together in our garden
Is where our contentment can grow.

I'm Hungry For You.

We may have different sexual appetites.
When it comes to eating in bed, there's different thinking:
Those who eat on the bed,
Or in the bed,
Or those who have the "no food in the bedroom" rule.

Usually those who have a television in their bedroom can relate to snacking
under the covers.
They recognize there's room for munchies
with the moves and grooves.

There are those who wish they could eat in the bedroom,
But their partner will have none of it.
They'll say, "No!" to the crackers, crumbs and crunchies.

When you get hungry,
You can always go to the kitchen,
Bring your talents to the table,
Turn up the heat,
Dish up some loving,
And get table laid.

I Haven't Had Sex For Such A Long Time; I Can't Remember The Last Time I Did.

Sometimes you have sex just because it's been too long.

You need some.
A reminder of when you did it all the time,
Or to refresh your memory of why you quit.

Sometimes all it takes is
To jump in the saddle,
To ride away,
To let your passions go,
To let loose,
To feel skin touching skin,
Feel the electricity,
Use it or lose it.

Have fun.
Find the right man or woman.
The one who turns you on.
And perform again.

You Have An Incredible Imagination.

You intrigue me.
Your energy,
Your ideas and methods,
You're full of surprises!

Ambiance,
Atmosphere,
Chemistry between us,
The light of the candles,
Music and nibbles,
Feeling the sensuality,
You're ready to try any position,
The blindfold,
The fantasy,
We laugh when we can't get it just right.

Variety is the spice of life.
You have the spice
And I want to taste it!

I Want To Continue The Journey With You.

You have goals and dreams, so do I.
You have a job and can contribute to our lifestyle.
You're dependable.
I think you'll make a good parent.
You're considerate.
You're kind to animals.
We can talk so easily about things.
We can disagree,
But we laugh about our differences.
We share the same values.
Your faith and spirituality is important.
You make me feel good about myself.
I want to reciprocate.

We're sexually compatible; it's a good fit.

This relationship is about liking me and loving my partner
We're different, but going down the same road.
My heart tells me that you're the one.
It will be a wonderful journey together.

I Want To Celebrate The Seasons Of Our Love.

Love is always in season.

Spring!
A seed of love is planted and we feel it grow.
A new beginning.
We encourage it to flourish and bloom,
A time to celebrate a new love.
Spring is when we're young at heart.

Summer!
A time to rest and appreciate.
We're in our prime.
We have the wisdom but we're still learning.
Summer is when we still have our energy.
We look to our future.

Fall!
A season when we're moving on in life.
A time to reflect on the years of accomplishments.
We've made adjustments.
Our roots are strong.
Our love has no age, and the best is yet to come.

Winter!
A season of contentment,
Of memories and shared experience.
We're so fortunate to make it to the winter of our lives.
Our love has truly been an incredible journey,
Which shall continue for as long as we both shall live.

To share the seasons of love,
Is truly a blessing.

I Want Revenge.

To get back at you,
To make you jealous,
To make you feel regret.
To make you think again.
To get you out of my system,
To know that someone else finds me attractive.

Two can play the game.

I've evened the score.
Pay back.

Revenge is mine.
Do I feel better now?

I Want To Take Care Of You.

To love you,
To understand you,
To help you deal with your complexities.

Some people are difficult.
They find it hard to get along.
They fumble with the right words.
They stumble through life.
Days can be difficult for them.

You've found each other and offer support.
To make a difference in your lives is a gift to one another.

To make a difference is not to try to fix or change someone,
But to stand by them, through thick and thin.
Through the ups and downs,
To help along the way,
To nurture,
To listen,
To find a better way,
Through patience and understanding,
Through love and compassion.

Everyone needs someone to love.

Never give up hope
Stay the course.
Give what you can during your time together.
Love is a gift to share and it comes back to you
In abundance.

I Want To Try Out My New Bed.

Buy a new mattress.
Firmer or softer.
Usually larger.

On average, mattresses last 10 to 15 years,
Depending on their quality
Or the quantity of work performed on them.

A new mattress may be the remedy for a squeaky bed.

Pay special care and attention to fancy sheets and pillows.
These are the ingredients to create the mood
For love and rest.
And you'll improve your pillow talk.
Your bedroom should be a central feature in your home.
Know that sleeping in separate beds can be lonely; attempt to work it out.

There's nothing like trying out a new mattress.
It's new!
A playground where it happens!

Have fun initiating it.
Slumber in your lover's arms.
Be a sleeping beauty,
And wake up with bed head.

I Feel Passion.
I Feel Lust.
I Feel Love.

We may certainly confuse lust with love,
But we recognize the differences
when we've experienced both.
Lust doesn't last but love certainly does.

Too often, when we're first experiencing sex,
It's about passion and lust.
We haven't yet grown into love.

Sex is about responsibility.
Sex should be safe, knowing your partner,
Practicing safe sex,
Using condoms—being safe, not sorry.
Talk to your doctor about birth control.
Talk to your partner about birth control.
It shouldn't be a taboo subject.

Who wants to face an unwanted pregnancy or disease?
It's a lousy feeling for the woman,
Counting the days until her period,
Worrying.
Think about changing the diapers, sleepless nights and the responsibility
of parenting.
It's about nervousness, waiting for the medical test results.
It's the long-term effects a disease may have on your health.
Go to the store and buy condoms—
You'll be glad you did in the morning.
(Parents shouldn't make young adults feel uncomfortable or guilty for
having condoms.)

Sex should be smart and safe.
Sex should be responsible.
Sex should be passionate.
Sex should be love.

You Are So Beautiful To Me.

I like what I see.
I like the way you make me feel.
Beauty is not only on the outside; it comes from within.

The reality is we can't always look our best.
There's garlic breath and morning breath.
There's bed hair and bad hair or no hair.
There are colds, flu, aches and pains.
There's growing old.
Add a few pounds here and there.
And cellulite.

There's the familiarity of our faces, as the hair turns grey,
And the wrinkles etched on our faces and bodies.

We need to look within.
As we go through the years creating memories
and living new experiences,
Our attachment goes beyond the physical beauty.
The emotional attachment and recollections create the glue keeping us
together.
We don't learn to love unless we share the experiences and appreciate each
other's inner beauty.

I love your special ways.
You turn me on, both inside and out.
You are so beautiful to me.

Sex Is Therapeutic.

Leave your troubles behind.
Find relief.
Escape together.
Share a bath.
Soap up in the shower.
Add candles, music, bubbles and fragrance,
Leather, lace, fur and feathers,
Body paint and erotic foods.
Dress up with costumes,
Role-play,
Spice it up,
Give it variety.
Bring something new and different, not the same old routine.
Be the one to initiate sex!

Change is possible, if you want it,
If you're determined.

Be young in spirit, young at heart.
Replenish your soul.
Recharge your batteries.
Keep the sexual side of your relationship steamy.
Give the gift of time for just the two of you.
Take time to undress each other.
Get naked and caress.
Share your emotions.
Sex burns calories.
Work up a sweat.
Make magic!

I Want To Go On A Picnic.

Share an erotic picnic—at home, in bed or in a special romantic setting.

There are many food treasures to bring along on a romantic escape (but watch those food allergies).
Foods can be an aphrodisiac and stimulant.
Foods are fuel to savor:

- blueberries
- strawberries
- whipped cream and toppings
- chocolate
- chocolate body paint
- honey and syrup
- juicy peaches
- a big banana
- champagne
- ice
- ice cream
- or a massage oil party for two.

Feed each other.
Have a body feast.
Make a mess.
Use your partner for a dinner plate.
Savor small bites,
Licks and nips,
Juicy and delicious,
Be the frosting on the cake.

Feast from the plate of love!

I Just Got Out Of Jail... Or It Seems That Way.

"I just got out of jail," is a line you hear in the movies, unless you're into criminals and bad guys.

But no one wants to be in prison.
Maybe you've been locked away for a while
in a bad relationship.
It doesn't have to be a life sentence you carry with you.
Don't become reclusive, reach out.
Talk about your feelings and sadness.
Don't conceal yourself in armor.

Seek someone who can help you leave a difficult relationship.

Later, you can seek new companionship.
You don't need to be lonely or afraid.
Get out there.
Things will change when *you* decide they should be different.
You can find someone who wants to share his or her life
with you.
Reach for new beginnings.

The fear you may feel of being alone will leave.
The emotional and physical security can be found.

There is no "get out of jail free" card.
You make the decisions.
Bad choices bring bad luck.
Good choices bring good luck.

I'm Stressed And Need A Release.

When you're stressed out perhaps the last thing you're thinking about is sex
But maybe that's exactly what you need.

Shopping doesn't gratify.
Eating chocolate doesn't quite satisfy.
A fast run or physical exercise won't do it.
Banging your head against the wall leaves you
bruised and dizzy.

The tension is too much.

Try sex –
Hard core and pounding,
Panting,
Moaning,
Sweating,
Pleasuring,
Taking control,
Turn up the heat,
Get on top,
Lusty sex,
The climax—let it go!
The release of all your troubles!

Relief.

I Just can't Stand It Any More.

If you've had sex before,
You recognize the pressure.

It's hard to explain.
It's hard to explain why you feel this way.
It's nature's way.
The sexual pressures build.
Sooner or later you just need some!

Yes, power tools are an option,
So is solo sex—your hands will do fine.
Yet the best is with a partner who wants to.

Enjoy the passion!

I'm Ovulating.

I think you'll make nice babies.
I want to have your baby.

What a terrific expression of love
To share a family,
A son,
A daughter,
A family,
Give the gift of life.

But don't pressure your partner,
You both need to be ready for this step.

Be prepared.
Sleepless nights,
Dirty diapers,
Someone who depends on you—totally!
Maturity is a must.
Responsibility is necessary.
Will your partner make a good parent?
How will you share the parenting responsibilities?
Sometimes a little one in need transforms us into a
good parent and a more mature adult.
Children take huge amounts of work and attention.
A life is depending on you.

If you're not ready for a baby in your life,
Use birth control.
If something unexpected happens,
Talk about your future.

You'll do just fine if you set your mind to it.

I'll Do Anything For A Fur Coat!

Most relationships offer one kind of trade off or another,
Whether you realize it or not.

It may be mowing the lawn, or taking out the garbage,
doing the dishes or maybe a treat after dinner.
It may be because you bring home the bacon
And your partner cooks it.
Or you make really good reservations at a restaurant.
For someone special,
You want to give the moon and the stars.
You worship the ground they walk on.

Relationships thrive on doing things for each other.
Rub my back.
Rub my feet.
Stay away from my feet.
Don't tickle my feet.
I'm not touching your feet.

Or, you can buy your partner something nice.
Surprise them.

When the trade is one way,
The relationship may lose its balance.

So barter or negotiate with your partner.

I'll make love to you if you buy me a fur coat .... (a faux fur will do).
Or, I'll make love to you if _____ (you fill in the blank)!

I Want To Have Lots Of Sex Before I Get Too Old.

Yes, our biological clocks are ticking, so enjoy it while you can.
Some are relieved when their partner's lost his or her MoJo....
You know, their libido.

Thanks to modern science, we have pills and thrills to motivate the lack luster.
If you have a low sex drive, go see your doctor.
Be honest in your discussions.
The pills may be just what you need.
You can be a love machine, once again.
Lotions and potions,
Lube and dube,
To slip and slide to sensuality.

If you're not into enhancements, good old physical activity and exercise
will work too.
Slow down on the booze and cigarettes.
Eat fruits and veggies,
Focus on improving your eating and physical habits.
That should rejuvenate your libido.

If, and when the day comes when you can no longer perform
Or deliver,
Or don't have the interest,
Remember that communication, laughter, understanding and compassion
With your companionship, affection and love
Will last a lifetime.

Our Relationship Smells Good.

The fragrance of a loved one lingers long after he or she is gone.
Isn't it memorable when you smell your date on your clothes?
On your skin?
You smell and remember....
The scent of love in the air,
Pheromones are working,
You want more.

The aroma of a sexy perfume or cologne,
The scent of someone fresh from the shower,
Smells good,
Looks good,
Don't hold back!

Smell can be powerful.
Your aroma will leave an impression.

I remember your scent,
And I want to see you again.

You Taste So Good.

The taste of you makes me hungry
And I'm not talking about food.
Remember our first French kiss?
The taste of sweat?
From your chest?
The taste of where only the brave will go.
The taste of your partner
Can drive you over the edge,
It will leave you hungry,
And wanting more.

This Song Puts Me In The Mood!

Music is a powerful stimulant to move you.
Groove together.
It sets the mood for romance.
Slow dance in the kitchen if you don't want to go out.

Remember special songs.
Memories from long lost lovers,
Or when you first met,
When you first made love….
A song that you share with your partner as "your song".

Set the mood with music.
Find your song together.
Feel the music in your heart.
Feel the rhythm.
Feel it….
In each other's arms.

I Need To Try Again; I've Lost At Love Once More.

Everything that happens to us
Is an opportunity to learn about ourselves.
Each experience tests our heart.
We may not know love until it's gone.
And then we understand.

We learn to love.

We can love many times in our life.
If it doesn't work out,
The experiences will lead us to our next love.

Each love touches our heart and makes its mark.
But it's our last love that is the most powerful,
The one that keeps us in love.

I Can't Sleep; I Need Sex.

I'm restless, tossing and turning.
I have a beautiful person lying beside me.
Your mind, body and soul arouse me.
I'm trying to go to sleep,
But I can't get you out of my mind.
I gaze at you in the morning light when you're sleeping.
I want to wake you.
I want you.
I nudge you, to get a response.
You continue to sleep.

So I let you slumber,
But I want sex ....
Later.

I'll try again,
Rest assured.

We're Finally Away On Vacation!

There's something to say about vacation sex.
Whether it's a weekend away or a long holiday,
Different surroundings,
Away from the pressures and everyday routine,

Vacations give you free time.
You're rested.

There's a problem though, if you're saving your sex
just for vacation,
If you're not careful, it will be a permanent vacation—
From each other.

Take a vacation and have sex in a strange bed!

I'm Drunk!

Sometimes alcohol can help with your mood.
Taste the spirits of whiskey and wine.
While a little liquor can loosen up the stress or routine, and give you courage,
it can also improve your mood.
But proceed with caution.

Too often, people may drown their sorrows, feeling lost and lonely or
thinking of lost loves.
Women who have been with drunk men, know all too well about
passed out passion.
Men who have been with women, know all too well about them passing out,
Or holding their heads as they vomit.
Too much drinking can mean alcoholism,
Doing things out of character.
It leads to regrets.
Being desperate means doing desperate things.

Being wasted isn't cool.
Alcoholics are lonely.
Alcoholism leaves you in depression.
Too much alcohol brings broken hearts and shattered dreams,
So can other addictions.

If you're suffering from any substance abuse,
Joint a support group.
Seek counseling and get help.
Kick the habit.

Once you come to your senses,
You'll know that drunken sex is poor sex.
It leaves a void.
Less is more when it comes to drinking.

Yet the reality is
Some of us have sex when we've had too much to drink.

You're So Sexy; You're So Hot!

Packaging makes a difference!

For her:
- a dress that fits perfectly,
- a thong and lacy bra,
- smooth and silky after a trip to the esthetician,
- show some cleavage, dab perfume in the hot spots,
- high heels,
- Adopt a classic look.

For him:
- shave the stubble and smell good,
- no saggy underwear with holes,
- if you've got way too much body hair, consider a wax job,
- no white socks unless you're wearing sneakers,
- toss the running shoes unless you're doing sports,
- Dress to impress.

Time to unwrap the package....
Let's undress and then
Wait for the reaction
And the action!

I'm In The Mood!

Your words are music to my ears.

Remember when you were always in the mood?

Let's keep that passion perking!
Maybe we need some life style changes?
Maybe I need to pay more attention?
Maybe I need to lay my hands on you with love pats and tender touches?
A date outside the house?
Footsies under the table?
Candlelight and music?

Compliment each other.
Talk about your dreams and accomplishments.
Be romantic.
Give lots of good hugs.
Physical and emotional attractions add up.
Attention to details count.
Showing you I'm committed to our relationship.

Sex just doesn't happen,
You have to create the moment.
It's the dividends of all you do.
Sex isn't always sensational,
Yes it changes.
Yet it can still be delicious.
Relationships aren't easy.
Relationships take time to create.
They require constant attention.

The mood just doesn't happen,
We have to create it—
Together.

You're My Fantasy.

Fantasies and dreams can become realities.

Someone special at work, at school,
You see them in your community.
They're on your mind.
Often.

You think about them,
And what might be.

Have courage, take a chance.
Don't be intimidated, have confidence.
Don't deny your hopes and dreams.
Have an open heart.
This is no time for relationship phobia.
Take a risk; you never know what will happen.

A smile, a few words or a touch
Can be the first step to beginning
A new relationship,
To companionship,
To a home,
To a family,
To a future of love and possibilities,
To make your dreams come true.

Be kind.
Be considerate.
But know when your advances may not be wanted.

Because I Love You.

The things we do for love—
Including giving sex—because we love our partner.

But there are times we just don't want to....
We're too tired.
We're hungry.
We're too busy.
We're achy.
We're moody.
We're sleepy.
It's too early.
It's late.
It's just not the right time.
You want to read your book.
You want to do your hair or nails.
Too much on our mind.
We're just not interested.
We procrastinate.

Sometimes we just go through the motions.
But it's important to be in the moment,
Not thinking about other stuff.

Give in.
Give it up.
We do it because we love our partner.

It's Time To Celebrate!

It's a home run.
You've crossed the finish line.
You've nailed it.
You've won the game!

Whether you're a player or fan,
Nothing captures the spirit more than a victory!

The emotion is extreme.
The play is energized.
It's exciting.
The energy of victory—
Celebrate with someone you love.
You've triumphed!

You've got endurance and stamina,
You're burning calories,
You feel the emotion.
Don't be a spectator,
Participate and enjoy the action!

Sex is a great sport.
Every time you make love,
Feel like a winner.
Be in the game!

And remember, in your relationship,
Don't keep a scorecard of who's right or wrong.

You've Caught My Attention.

We make eye contact;
There's something between us.
We're giving off the right signals to each other—
A connection.

From the first moment, you took my breath away.
My heart is pounding.
My emotions are stirring.
I feel awkward.
I may not say the right words.

I just have to get to know you.
Be brave, ask the question:
Would you like to go for coffee?
A movie? A dance?
Exchange numbers or email addresses?
Agree to see each other again?

Believe in love.
Believe in yourself.
Believe in love at first sight.
Believe in head-over-heels love.

Look to the future.

I Don't Want To Miss A Day Loving You.

Once an emotional bond of love and passion takes hold,
The senses take over.

When love and sex is new,
It's so powerful that you think of nothing else.

You do live on love, in the beginning.

Is it the sex you love?
Or is it the person you love to have sex with?

Only when the sex cools off can you figure it out.

You turn my head.
You turn me on.
I long for you,
Your fragrance,
The color of your hair,
The sparkle in your eye,
The way you touch me,
The way my heart skips,
The way you kiss,
Your compassion,
Your strength.
Sharing with each other
The good and not so good.

But most of all,
You love me too.

I Love Morning Sex.

A great way to start the day.
A kiss in the morning,
Even with morning breath or angel's breath.
You stroke me gently, a nudge, a caress,
A whisper of endearments,
Not choosing sleep over sex.
Early morning luvin!
A fantastic way to start the day off right!

Some like to sleep in late,
Others are early risers,
It helps if you're both morning people.
But what's important ….
Don't sleep through your relationship.

Smile,
If you've had morning sex.

I Need The Practice.

When you first start out,
You may feel like you're lost in the woods.
Awkward moments:
You're shy,
You don't know what to try,
You're fumbling for the buttons,
Are you hitting the right spot?

Have some nerve.
Laugh together.
Find your funny bone and laugh at yourself.
Have a tickle.
Do what comes natural.
Don't be afraid to talk during sex.
Let your partner know what you like
And what you don't like.
Don't be shy.
Be uninhibited;
Experiment.
Practice makes a good lover,
Along with giving your compassion, respect, concern, unselfishness,
patience and humor.

Talk to each other,
And listen with your heart.
Explore and discover.
You'll find each other.
You'll be good lovers.

Experience is the best teacher.
And practice makes perfect.

Have Sex For Old Time's Sake.

Your paths cross again.
Seeing an ex.
You remember the old flame.

But sometimes it's just that....
An old flame.
Only a flicker.
The embers will not burn again.

Sex for old time's sake
Can be a huge mistake.
Think about it.

And other times
It can be reignited
To a new, rekindled burning blaze.

How will you know?

It's My First Time And I Want It To Be With You.

This reason may sound like a line, but it's true.
You're nervous, not knowing what to expect.
The first time can be scary, traumatic, eventful, memorable, and spectacular—all in one—
Or disastrous.

The first time can happen because
You're in love, in lust or just plain infatuated—
Or, you just want to get it over with.

Don't have performance anxiety during your first time,
Enjoy the experience.

You're vulnerable.
Your first one should be with someone you love,
And someone you trust.
It shouldn't be something you regret.

Virginity can never be taken back.
Choose carefully.

I Want To Share My Fantasy And It's Fun To Dress Up.

It's Halloween, and time for a treat!

Halloween is the perfect time to buy new costumes,
Like the French maid,
Or your super Hero!
Be rock stars!

There's the fantasy of a nurse dressed in white,
Do a checkup on your sex life.
Be a bunny with fishnet stockings and a corset,
Playboy ears and tail can be a turn on.

But if she doesn't like spiders, Spiderman is the wrong choice.
Maybe Superman can take her to new heights!

If it doesn't work out,
At least you'll have a great laugh together!
Or you'll have a great memory of seeing your partner in a new way!
As you try to spice up your relationship.

Want more passion?
Share your fantasies!

It's The Holiday Season For Us.

A time to give and a time to receive.
A time to exchange your presents,
And your presence.

Or, it's Boxing Day.
Or, it's New Year's Eve.

Maybe the family was around too much during the
holiday season.
Maybe you were too tired because of the holiday hustle
and bustle.

Seek an alternative time to honor the box on Boxing Day!
Get ready for the New Year.
Create your own fireworks!

Because It's Earth Day.

April 21st each year.

It's the day to do it

- on the green grass,
- in the wilderness,
- under the clouds,
- on a mountain,
- in the fresh air,
- on the beach,
- while skinny dipping,
- after fishing for trouser trout,
- while feeling the sun's energy.

Pay tribute to Mother Earth.
Nature is a beautiful place.

Have great sex.
Feel the Earth move,
And go organic!

I Feel Sexy In My New Underwear.

You'll like what I'm wearing!

Purchased any new sexy undergarments lately?

No one likes baggy or saggy or discolored ginch.
No one likes stretched out or discolored panties.
Try a thong – you might like it.
Say goodbye to granny panties.
Once a year, out with the old and in with the new
When it comes to under garments.

New underwear can give you that extra confidence and spring in your step!
Even though no one can see them,
You know you have it!
Confidence and sex appeal.
Whether you roar it up with animal prints, racy red, sexy black or puritan white,
You'll see it and your partner will see it.
You feel it working.

Go commando,
Or choose boxers or briefs.
Men, don't have prettier lingerie than your women.

The unexpected is a terrific surprise.

Remember the real reason to wear nice underwear...
Is not because a bus may hit you,
It's because you may get lucky!

You Look So Sexy

You're hot!

Foxy and looking good,
Fashionable,
Not frumpy,
A mind and a body,
A classic and seductive beauty,
Alluring,
Luscious lips,
An extra spritz of perfume,
A thong,
Or no thong.

For the man;
Clean,
No body odor,
A manicure,
Boxers or briefs,
Pressed, not wrinkled,
Good shoes,
Smelling good but not too strong,
Good conversationalist,
A smile and charisma to close the deal.

You are what you think.
Have a positive self-image.
No grilling and no interrogation,
Interesting discussions,
A good listener,
Your confidence is inviting.

Be hot!
You're hot!
Why not?

I Love Calling You By Your Pet Name.

It's that special secret between us.

I have a special name for you.
Pet names....
They're fun and loveable.

Bubbles, Cupcake, Sweet pea, Pooh Bear, Sunshine,
Sugar Pie, Sugar Buns, Sugar Beet, Sugar Plum, Sunflower, Honey Bun,
Honey Pot, Honey Dew, Sweetheart, Princess, Queenie, Angel, Darling,
Lovey, My Love, Peaches, Sweetums, Beaver, Jewel, Sapphire, Foxy, Baby
Cakes, Poppy, Jellybean.

Or

Stud, Steamer, Superman.
Jackhammer.

What you don't want to use is
My old Lady, or
My old Man.

Once your friends find out your pet name
Its special meaning is lost.

Know that once you choose a pet name,
Be careful.
It sticks forever.

You're My Best Friend.

I've looked in the bars,
I've checked out singles dating,
I've been in the chat room,
I've played the matchmaker's game,
I've used the dating services.

I'm looking for someone special;
Someone who can be my lover and my best friend.

Maybe you've looked too far
And what you're looking for is very near.
Your best friend may be someone with whom you have a comfortable
friendship,
But you haven't taken it to the next step.
How would you feel if your best friend was getting married?

Maybe you want to take it to the next level.
See what develops,
Perhaps intimacy?

Best friends can be forever.

I'm Lonely; I Need Someone.

To walk alone is lonely,
To sleep alone is cold.

We all want someone to share our lives with.

There's a difference between being alone and being lonely.
Learn to enjoy your own company first, and being alone.
Then you'll appreciate the closeness,
And the companionship will complete you.

Someone to fill your time and space,
To share your secrets,
To share your hopes and dreams,
To hear music and dance together,
To converse and connect.
To be best friends.

You can sit in silence
Together.
And understand each other and say,
"I'm not lonely anymore!"

I'm Ready To Have Sex—Again.

You're up for it almost all the time.
Where do you get your sex drive?
You're insatiable.
Your desire is a turn on.
You have an incredible libido.

I can have sex whenever I want!

The desire between us is magic.

Who can keep up with the pace?
If you're grumbling about too much sex,
Remember,
Age catches up with us.
The passion may diminish.
Eventually hot cools down.

Enjoy it while it lasts!

Shopping Is A Turn-on.

It's a sport for most women.
Gotta love those fashionistas and shopaholics!

Most women like to shop more than men.
For most men, shopping is a chore;
It's not a pleasurable outing or experience.
Know that retail therapy works wonders for women – it gives a high!
That includes shoe shopping for those who have a
passion for shoe fashion!

Shopping for something sexy.
Or just window-shopping.

Shopping together can be an adventure.
Let your partner know how much you enjoy
his or her company during your shopping adventure.
"Come with me into the dressing room
while I try on the lingerie…."

Shopping can be a trade off.
Shopping first; sex later.

Bring your credit card.
A shopping treat for a sex treat!

I Need Help To Get Over Someone.

Sometimes we need a new relationship
To help us get away from a bad one.
If you keep thinking about the past,
You may lose out on your future.

Whether beginning a new relationship
Or ending your relationship,
It can be hard to make a break.
But another person can help us move forward.
Someone new can be a stepping-stone into the future.

A new relationship helps us make a clean break,
Rather than staying in an unhealthy one.

Yes, it's difficult to make the first step and walk away.
Without someone new, we may return to the familiar,
former relationship.
It's troubling and isn't good for us.
We know it,
Deep down.

We stay in an unhealthy relationship just because it's someone,
And we don't want to be alone.
Remember that being alone and unhappy
Is better than being with someone and unhappy.
If you leave, it's short-term pain for long-term gain.
So the relationship didn't survive, but you do,
And you're better for it.

Some of us make the transition between relationships
better than others do.
If you can, re-establish yourself first, emotionally and mentally.
Don't go into the next relationship when you're vulnerable.

Don't be afraid to be alone.
Move on when you're ready.

Now That I've Gotten To Know You, You're So Much More Than What I Expected.

We all have prejudices and biases.
We may think differently or react to people because of their job, their background, the color of their hair, or the way they dress….
Or worse, because of their race, nationality, sexuality
or disability.

What's important is that we become aware of our prejudices,
And we become tolerant and accepting,
And open-minded to differences.

Tolerance and acceptance is a gift we give to others,
And to ourselves.
Accepting differences is important in a relationship.

You may be surprised,
Once you get past your intolerance or narrow mindedness.

It will be so much more than you imagined.
You'll be a better person.

I Feel Sexy, I Feel Young!

It's all about attitude!

It happens…you wake up and fear losing your desirability.
You're no longer eye candy or you no longer turn heads.

So you get a little help.
No matter what your treatment—Botox or surgery,
You can feel good about yourself,
It's self-improvement on the outside,
Because our body image has so much to do with our
inner confidence.

Balding men can be sensitive about their thinning hair,
And losing their hair.
But the man who feels confident in his body and skin, is attractive.
You're only old if you think you're old.

Frumpy, dumpy and lumpy isn't appealing or attractive—
to you or your partner.
Work out, get some physical exercise, look your best.
Make good food choices.
When you look good, you feel good!

Don't begrudge those who get Botox, or a nip and a tuck.
Or those who rely on hair dye.
They're not vain.
They're growing old in their way,
Or renewing themselves.
They feel good, again.

Whatever you choose, over time,
With or without the lights is still an option,
You always look good in the soft and dim light.

Learn to love and appreciate yourself.
Celebrate your beauty and your body at any age!
And remember, never wear a flannel nightie or long johns unless you're sick
or it's minus thirty below!

Your Seduction Is Working.

Your flirting is enchanting me;
You've wrapped me around your finger.

You're driving me crazy;
I'm filled with lust and my desire is stirring.

It's the tease,
The tantalizing,
The chase,
The ritual of romance,
The come on,
A wink,
The look,
A nod or tilt of the head,
A smile,
A touch,
A compliment,
Your smell,
The contours of your body,
It's seduction through the senses.

Take a chance,
Introduce yourself,
Begin the dance to romance.

Seduction usually means action.
Take a chance....
It starts with hello.

I Want To Make It Up To You.

We all make mistakes through actions or words.

Nattering about the quirks or little things about your partner.
In the beginning, might be fun and humorous.
But if the words continue, it becomes a bad habit.
What once was clever is now hurtful.
Be sensitive, not sarcastic.

Be careful of words you can never take back.
Be remorseful.
Apologize, and mean it.
You can't rewind the tape, once it's said.
Words can wound.
Keep anger in check.
Tame your temper and get a handle on your hostility.
Chill.
If you've forgotten an important date,
A missed anniversary or special occasion,
Or if you've said or done something that's hurtful,
Or bruised the relationship,
Take time to make amends.

"I'll make it up to you," are important words.
"I'm sorry," are healing words.
Do what it takes to repair the damage.
Make-up sex is grand—
You both win.

I'm Attracted To The Young Stuff.

But not to jailbait.

Some women love the young guys.
Their appetite for sex is exhausting and incredible.
But hard male bodies.
May love you and leave you.

Some young men appreciate the sophistication
of an older woman.
But be cautious, they may be looking for a mother.

Then there's the older man and the younger beauty;
Do you want a nurse or a purse (preferably with assets)?
Are you sure you can keep up?
Slow down, you may have a heart attack.

What about marrying someone ten years younger?
If you're a woman, and have a younger partner –
You'll feel younger,
And keep your youth longer.
If you're a man, you'll always have someone to look after you and tend to
your needs.
You may not have the six-pack abs anymore
But you'll have the trophy on your arm.

Having a content partner—no matter what the age—
Is the best accessory you can have.

When the novelty wears off these romances,
You take with you the memories
And an appreciation of the love and passion.

And, if you're lucky, you grow old together.

I Need Someone To Show Me The Way.

I'm young, confused and don't know enough.

Maybe someone with more experience
Can give me a few hints.
You're inexperienced,
You're keen and interested.

You can rent a movie,
Purchase a "how to" book,
Learn bedroom skills together,
You can be honest with what you like,
And what you don't like.
You can experiment together.

All sex acts may not be for you.

Be sensitive and caring,
Talk about what you like
And what you don't like.
Explore together.
Let nature take its course.
You'll find your sexual way.

Because It's Raining.

Unless you go walking in the rain, what else can you do
when it's grey and wet outside?

A good time to—
Build a fire,
Run a bath,
Make the mood hot,
Have a drink to warm your spirit,
Cuddle in the blankets.

Those wet spring and summer rains make things fresh,
They wash away the dust in our lives.

When you see clouds, don't think about the blues,
Because, before you can have rainbows, you need the rain.

Find the pot of gold together!

I'm Having A Party!

Come on over,
I'm having a party.
Parties capture the mood of flirting,
Excitement,
Lust, and
Maybe, the beginning of love.

Just as good food is all about the presentation,
So too, are appearance and atmosphere—the keys for ambience.

Dress up.
Be noticed.
Light the candles.
Music sets the mood.
Pour a drink.
Find a corner or a closet,
Sneak away for a quick one.
Party sex makes a great memory!

If you get caught,
You'll be the talk of the town.

You Make Me Feel Alive!

We can go through life living each day,
Until the moment when you meet someone who sparks you,
Makes you look again,
Makes your heart warm.
You feel alive.
You've met your match and
The one you've been searching for.

The thrill of love is in the air.
You've found what you're looking for.
You find yourself smiling and dancing!
You sail through the day to be with the one you love.
Chemistry.
The potion of love.

If you're lucky in love.
Once is enough.

We Have The Right Chemistry.

It's magnetic attraction.
When you look at that person,
You just know.

We send out messages,
And when the signals are returned,
It's magic,
It's desire,
It's a connection.
You have lots in common.
You're both available.

Chemistry and connection is important.
It doesn't happen with everyone you meet,
So when you feel it,
Act upon it!

I'd Like To See If I Can Get You In My Bed.

It's a test to see if you like me enough
To give yourself to me.

A notch in the belt for the man.
A note in the journal for the woman.

Beware of the smooth ones who always know what to say.
You respond to the move, the hustle, and the tease,
But don't be a pushover.

It's a great feeling when your advances are rewarded.
But when you're rejected, it hurts.

But don't take rejection to heart,
It just wasn't meant to be.
There's another challenge, another encounter,
Waiting to happen.

But on the other hand, if you like hot and steamy sex,
And you're not afraid of a one-night stand,
Go for it.
Have fun.
You'll have some great flashbacks and memories!
But don't forget to practice safe sex.

I Missed You.

You've been away for a while.
The place is not the same without you.

I miss the comfort of your arms,
Your smile, your scent, the warmth of your body
When we lay down at night.

But most of all
I miss you.
You soothe my soul.
You comfort me.

The anticipation of seeing your lover
After a time apart
Can be exciting.
Suppressed sexual desire can overflow.
Absence makes the heart grow fonder.
Keep in touch.
Connect by phone.
Yes, you can always try phone sex.
Phone sex is safe sex.
Your lover's voice can heat up your loins or the phone lines!

But nothing is better than skin to skin,
Holding each other again.

It's Grandpa's And Grandma's Birthday.

An old timer was asked on his birthday
Whether he would like super-sex.
He heard soup or sex.
He said, "I'll take the soup."*

When you get older, you don't need a reason.
You just hope it works.

Grandmas and Grandpas need luvin' too.
And if you're retired,
You definitely have the time.

*author unknown

You're A Generous Person.

Some people are begrudging with their time.
Tight-fisted with their money.
Sparing with their love.
They lack the spirit of generosity.

It's been said, there are two kinds of people.
Givers
And
Takers.

Givers are generous,
Kind hearted,
Gentle spirits,
Easier to love,
Always there.

Takers sit back and watch it happen.
They get upset when things aren't going their way.
They have a tough outer shell.
They need attention.
Emotionally, takers can drain you.

Be a giver,
Work at it.

You'll reap the rewards of a generous heart.

I'm Taking A Chance On Love.

The stakes are high in any relationship.
You've opened your heart and you are vulnerable.

It's the relationship that matters the most.
Be good friends.
Be lovers and
Work at it day by day.

When the sex slows down, you'll have each other,
Along with the hugs and companionship.
Sharing and growing together.

It's been said that the best relationships are like a tree:
They provide shelter, but
Are strong enough to bend, and
Provide protection during tough times.

Be like the tree as your love grows,
And over the years, develop long, deep roots that
grow and strengthen.

Taking a chance is worth it.

I Sleep So Much Better After Sex.

It's been a long day.
You've been on my mind.
My emotions are intense,
The pressure is building,
I need the release,
I need to feel you.

Let me show you my love and passion.
Undress seductively and slip between the sheets.
We lie together,
Feeling the warmth,
Your fingers touch me,
And excite me,
Caressing and kissing,
Reaching the peak!
Relaxed—
What a wonderful way to end or begin our day.

And I'll sleep so much better after sex.

It's Your Turn To Get On Top!

We take turns—who gets on top.
We're not just talking about the bedroom.

Relationships should not be competitive, but cooperative.
In fact, too much competition between each other
Can cause friction.
Competition is usually about winning and losing.
Competition can bring about tensions between each other.
Competition can hurt each other's feelings.

Try cooperation instead.
Cooperation is about helping each other
Giving and taking,
Reaching goals,
And sharing accomplishments.
Cooperation achieves
And brings better results in a relationship.
Cheer each other on instead of proving who is better.
Have concern for the other's person's feelings.

Try cooperation instead of competition.

Who is the dominant one in your relationship?

Take turns being on top.
Try a new position.

You're What I'm Looking For In A Woman.

You're strong but not overbearing.
You're gentle, nurturing and sensitive.
Your touch, your concern, your compassion,
You're there when I need you,
The way you walk, talk, and stimulate my mind
Is what I'm looking for.

You say you can change a tire,
But you have the number of the towing company, just in case.

You're not afraid to put on your boots and show me
What you're made of—
A combination of the girl next door and my erotic dream.
You know enough about sports to converse about the game.
You can have a drink, but you know your limit.

You watch the make over shows,
But don't try to make me over.

You get an "A" in domestic responsibilities.
You've shared your home-making skills with me,
And have taught me there is a male role to play
in our household.
You make a nice bed and a comfortable home.

You check out the male muscles and abs,
But always say you prefer my body.

After all the years, you still turn me on.
I can't stop loving you.
And most of all, you love me too.

You're What I'm Looking For In A Man.

Your masculinity is strong
But you're in touch with your feminine side.
You not only like to cook,
But you like to watch the cooking shows.
And you cook in the bedroom too!

You like to go shopping and buy things for our home,
You'll hold my purse and not be embarrassed.

You like to watch the decorating shows—for a while.
You wait until they are finished until you change
To the sports channel.

You're strong, physically and emotionally.
I feel safe with you.
You have a good soul.

You let me drive,
And don't get pissed if we have to stop for directions.

And while I occasionally catch you checking out
The women on the street,
I don't get upset or envious.
Your head always turns back to me.
After all these years, you say I'm still a knockout.

We've hit the ball out of the ballpark.
It's a homerun for our relationship.

I'm Willing To Commit.

I'm willing to walk down the aisle with you.

I'm willing to give up my freedom and share new beginnings.
I'm afraid of the unknown.
But I choose love.

There comes a time when we're ready;
Ready for the commitment based on our judgment,
Based on our emotions,
Based on the dreams I want to share with you.
My heart is telling me,
The time is right.

I'll put my heart on the line.
Wild horses can't drag me away from you.

I have your name written on my heart.
I'm ready to commit.

I believe happily ever after, can happen with you.
Along with our love,
It takes commitment and work.

Your Tattoo Intrigues Me.

Where do I find it?

The choice of a tattoo says a lot,
So does the location.
Some show them off.
Others have them in discreet locations.
Tattoos can be intriguing.

How low does it go?
Downtown or on the behind?
To search and seek is part of the adventure!

Tattoos make a statement,
It's an identification mark,
An expression of individuality.

Maybe there's a piercing that can be a surprise too!

I'll show you mine if you show me yours!

Surprise!

I Want To Help Heal Your Scars.

You can share some of you and I'll share some of me,
But I'm thinking that you hide your scars well.

Some of us have emotional scars.
We don't want to talk about our past,
Bad memories,
Bad feelings,
Bad experiences.
Some hang-ups we need to get over,
Scars on the outside,
Scars on the inside.

You can open up to someone and tell your stories.
You make the decisions to begin to heal,
Or you can keep your secrets and learn to live with your hurts.

We all have scars—some have more than others.
It's how we wear them that counts.

You Won't Be Seeing Me For A While,

I'm going on a trip.

Goodbye sex.
It can be bittersweet,
Melancholy,
Not knowing when you'll next see,
And feel each other.

Time apart….
Distance in the relationship,
Or a long drive to see each other.

Love gives you strength.
You will go through great lengths to love again
And see each other.
Distance is a formality.
Time apart—it's worth waiting for your return.

Until we meet again,
I'll think of you so often.

You Make Me Laugh!

What a hoot! What a laugh!
I didn't know it was that small.
It's how you use it that counts!
I'm sorry I laughed.
It's not that small, after all!

A good laugh and humor in a partnership
Goes a long way.
Laughter is great medicine,
Or an icebreaker.
An aphrodisiac for the ears—
Creating a mood altering moment.

The funny guy doesn't always get the girl,
But it's a great way to try.

To bring a smile, be yourself.
Go easy on the questionable or bad taste jokes.
Bringing humor to the relationship is not about
Being the centre of attention.
Go for a giggle,
Laughter can brighten one's day and night,
To fill the room with cheer,
And mega smiles.

Plus, a happy person is appealing.

I Feel The Music And I Want To Dance With You!

Sex is like dancing, you have to know the moves:
Samba, merengue, cha-cha,
Two-step, polka, fox trot, the waltz, the jive, the twist!
The dirty dog,
Hip-hop,
Rock 'n roll,
Salsa dancing,
Let's twist and shout,
Or just move and groove.

Women love men who are willing and ready to dance.
It's romantic to dance together.
And, there's nothing like a slow dance
When I can feel you against me.

So dance with me,
Share the rhythm,
Share the music.
It takes two to tango and,
You've danced your way into my heart.

I Really Know You.

When a couple's been together for a while,
They begin to know each other's signals.
A look across the room,
A gesture,
A smile, a wink—the look.

Laughing at the same old jokes—
Knowing when it's time to leave the party.

It's the familiarity that makes it comfortable.

The touch of a loving hand,
Knowing the expression in your eyes,
The sound of your voice when you're up and you're down,
The awareness of each other's signals,
Whether intentional or not.
It's one of the great rewards of a long-term relationship.

I know you,
And it's good.

We've never lost that honeymoon feeling!

I Need Satisfaction.

To see you satisfied,
To see that smile on your face,
To watch your expression of passion,
To see the look of love in your eyes.

Love is a demonstrative experience.
It's not enough to say the words;
You need a loving touch and caress,
A kiss on the cheek,
A nibble to be naughty,
A back rub, a foot massage,
Helping around the house,
Kind words and respect,
Affection,
Humor.

It's a partnership where both contribute.
To do the best you can
To achieve personal and couple satisfaction.

That is success.

I Caught You!

I caught you doing it on your own.
You look so satisfied.
Let me help you with that!

If you're lonely and by yourself,
Hands on,
Or sex toys,
Work fine.

But with me around,
You don't have to do it alone.
If you need more,
Let me know,
Let me watch.
Don't be scared to ask for what you need.

Now and then,
You may need a little in between,
On your own,
But don't make a habit of it.

It's better with the two of us!

We've Been Together; It's Time For More.

Let's test the waters and live together.
Let's take the next step.
Let's learn even more about each other.
And if it works out, the next step is marriage.
Days and nights, we share more.
We'll have a sense of belonging.
The value placed on marriage,
Two can live cheaper than one.
If it doesn't work out, we can both walk away.
Without the hassle of a divorce.

Or should it be marriage?
We'll get all of the above,
Along with the blessings and a marriage certificate.

Some of us are comfortable and more than happy
To live together
Without the formality of marriage.
Others may have a difference of opinion on marriage
And agree or disagree,
On what's next in the relationship.

Don't automatically lose someone special if they won't commit to marriage.
Work it out.
There's a lot to debate.

Either way, it's serious.
It's called commitment.
There's a decision to make—
Together.

I Love You, Just The Way You Are.

You have my heart.
With love and adoration,
Our love is giving and sharing.

I see the sparkle in your eye.
I feel your smile.

Our senses are in sync.
We know each other well.
 I sense your passions and desire.
Your emotions stir me.

This relationship is the best I've ever had.
A kiss every day for the rest of our lives.
My heart is yours—
Yesterday, today and tomorrow.

We can't change each other.
We can only change ourselves.
I love you, for who you are,
Not who I want you to be.

& Just As Many Reasons Not To

You're Too Materialistic For Me.

In our pursuit of happiness, perhaps we fill our life
With too much stuff.

Our true needs are few, yet our wants are many:
The elegant home, expensive furniture, the fast car, the fancy clothes and
the glitzy bling—
Huge mortgage,
Maxed credit cards,
Car payments,
School fees,
Bills, bills and more bills,
We're buried in debt.
We're feeling overwhelmed.
No room to breathe.

Financial stress can ruin one's sex life.
So can too much clutter in the relationship.

Is there enough room for my needs and for me?

I want love and inner calm,
You have escalating demands,
And always want more.
Your world and my world just don't mesh.

I Need To Solve My Problems First.

At the many stages of our lives, we all have luggage.

The question is – how much do we have?

A small carry on? A few suitcases? Trunks full?
How do you carry your luggage?

Analyze what happened in past relationships.

What went wrong?
Why wasn't I fulfilled?
What role did my partner play?
What role did I play?

Don't bring your old problems into a new relationship.
Don't piggy back old problems onto new problems.
Get rid of any anger, hostility or resentment you may feel.
Let it go.
Forgiveness of yourself and others, frees you from anger and bitterness.

Experience can be a valuable teacher
As long as we learn from it.
Improve yourself daily.
Life may not work out the way we plan it or want it to be.

You can be the hero of your story,
Or the victim.
It's up to you—you choose.

Resolve your problems as much as you can,
So you're able to carry your own luggage.

You're Too Complicated.

You analyze this,
You evaluate that,
You think too deep,
You have to get to the root of the problem,
You have to fix everything,
And it has to be just right.
You border on perfection,
Your obsession is annoying.

To analyze a relationship to the core
Can be exhausting.
Lighten up!

There's nothing wrong with critical thinking,
But when it gets to the point of irritation,
And getting on your partner's nerves,

It's time to analyze yourself—
Not your partner,
Not the relationship,
You!

I'm PMS-ing.

It's a woman thing—
Pre-menstrual-syndrome.

For men, PMS may mean
Pretty-much-sexless.

Women can feel lousy:
Headache, bloating, unattractive, irritable and moody....

Or
They may have a spurt of sexual drive that's incredible!
Horny times!

But more often than not, pms-ing
Means *going without.*

I Don't Want To Do This Again.

Don't let history repeat itself.
Don't bring your old problems into a new relationship.
Solve the puzzles first, before you move on.

We can be attracted to the same character type,
Again and again.
Sometimes the qualities that you're attracted to in a person
Are the demise of a relationship later on.

You do a repeat – looking for the same kind of lover.
Sometimes they're too ambitious,
Too spontaneous,
Too independent, or
Too much of a social butterfly.
And you're the homebody, quiet type.
There are just too many different habits or traits
That isn't quite for you.

Find someone who complements your character and lifestyle.
Yes, opposites do attract,
But familiarity can bring contentment.

You Said You'd Call And You Didn't.

Nothing is more upsetting than when
You say you'll call and you don't.

If you're not interested, don't b. s.
Don't lead me on.
It hurts when you build false expectations.
Saying "I'll call you" and you don't
Is a kiss off phrase.

Instead, be honest;
It's the best practice.
It's okay, to let someone know you're not into them.
"I really don't think we have a connection but it was nice talking to you,"
will work just fine.
A blow off isn't considerate.

Don't stay home and wait for the call.
Go out and do something.
Become the best person you can be.

If they're really interested, they'll call
And make the connection.

I'm Cynical About Love.

I've had too many disappointing relationships.
My heart is bruised and hardened.
I've been used,
Abused,
Stepped on and discarded.
I've been dumped too many times.
I'm emotionally wounded.

To be cynical means you've closed your heart
To people
And opportunities to love.

Sometimes love is trial and error,
And you need to keep trying until you get it right.

While you're fragile, keep believing that you can trust again.

Your heart will love again.

I'm Tired Of Begging For It.

Like a dog waiting for a bone.

I'm like a puppy drooling,
Doing tricks.
Give me a treat,
I'll do something for you!

I'll buy you a present.
I'll rub your back.
I'll be really, really good.
I'll talk nice.
I'll make you supper.
I'll deliver breakfast in bed.
I'll take you away for a get-away.
I'll be good.
I'll do anything….

Enough already!
Give this dog a bone….

I Look At You And I'm Not Attracted To You Anymore.

We've been together for a while now.
I look at you and where is the appeal?
Where's the spark?
Are we both disinterested?
Have you let yourself go?

What happened to the good old days when we
Laughed, loved and lived happier times?
What happened to our bond and attraction?
Where did it go?

Yes, physical attraction is important to me,
But I feel I'm losing our emotional bond.
And my devotion to you.

We can't live in the past.
We have to move forward.
We can't ignore this.
We need to remember for better or for worse.

How do we get out of the rut we're in?

We could try counseling.
We could sit down and talk honestly about how we're feeling.
We can work towards a better *you*,
A better *me*,
And a better *us*.

We can't expect immediate results,
It will take time, love and patience.

I'm willing, are you?

You're Not Rich Enough For Me.

It's not shallow to want good things in life.
I want the lifestyle.
I want someone to take care of me.
I don't want to work.
I want to be kept.

I can be a Trophy Wife,
Or a Mr. Mom.

I think I can find someone wealthy and someone to love.
Some people call me a gold digger.

Show me the money and I'm yours!

Fine dining, fragrances,
Fancy digs, fine furniture,
Sports car, swimming pool,
Spa days,
So many vacation days....
No sorrows.

You can have a lot of money,
You can spend a lot of money.
It's not always easy to reach agreement
on how to spend the money,
But if you're not laughing or smiling in the inside,
There's something missing that you just can't purchase.

On second thought,
Maybe one shouldn't marry just for the money,
You'll end up paying for it—
One way
Or another.

Money can buy you sex and lifestyle,
But it can't buy you love.

I'm Not Making That Same Mistake.

I wish I knew then what I know now.

We cannot erase our past,
But we can learn from it.
Experience is the teacher.
Wisdom is what we get when we learn from our mistakes.

Don't make the same mistakes over and over.
Don't repeat bad history.
Don't be afraid to take risks.
Don't become cynical about love.
Even if you have a calloused heart.
Try again.

Growing and learning from
Our mistakes bring us to the lessons learned.

We all have them.

Your Personality Is Prickly.

When we first met, I thought there was an attraction.

But as I got to see the real you I'm disillusioned.
I'm disappointed.
Now you're showing the real you.

How you talk to the servers in the restaurant,
How you treat the clerk in the store,
How you speak to your mother and father.
Your aggression when driving,
Your lack of generosity,
The occasions when you whine,
Your tendencies to be dominating and too controlling,
A hidden anger that lashes out unexpectedly,
At times, you're cold and standoffish—
You have that "all about me" syndrome.

I'm seeing a different side.

We're not compatible.
I enjoy the simplicity in life.
I want fewer things and more substance;
Having a partner that loves me as I am.
Having a partner that thinks *we*, not *me*.
That's the wealth of the relationship I'm looking for.

We're definitely different;
We're not a match.

I'm glad I see it now, rather than later on in our relationship.

I Don't Want To.

Before you go out on a date,
Or during other occasions in your life,
Be prepared and be able to say:

- No
- No Sir
- No Miss
- No thank you
- Not now
- Not ever
- I'm not ready
- I don't want to
- No way
- No guilt

Practice saying "no."

Do the role-playing
Whether it's a mover or a shaker,
A friend that's putting the make on you,
A head turner that makes you think twice,
Someone making you feeling guilty,
Just say, "no!"
Not on the first date....

Be strong,
Know what you want.
Don't succumb to peer pressure.
It's okay to be celibate.
Abstinence from sex is just fine.

Sex is a gift to give of your choosing.
You don't need to argue.
You don't need to debate.
You have the right to refuse.

No sex at this time of your life.
Just say "no" if you're not ready.

Something Is Wrong.

I don't know what it is.
It's a feeling in my heart,
That gut feeling,
In my stomach,
In my mind….
The intuition….
A rush of emotion not to go there.

Yes, I'm lonely,
But I'm not sure about you.
Maybe I should take a chance?
I feel so many emotions right now.

But it just doesn't feel right.
First impressions can be instinctive;
Trust them,
Trust your intuition.

When in doubt, don't.
Live to love another day.

It's Valentine's Day And It Sucks.

I'm lonely.
I have no one to have sex with.

Some people will dump their partner before Valentine's Day.
They can't handle the pressure of the relationship,
They want to avoid the commitment,
the gift or the expectations.

What do you do when you don't have a Valentine?

Don't worry.
It can be an overrated holiday.
The chocolate is fattening.
The flowers wilt.
Too many line-ups at the restaurants.
You'll save money.
Cupid's arrow hasn't struck you yet.

You're still searching for the love of your life.

It's not your turn.
Maybe next year.

I'm Not Ready.

I'm just not ready to be intimate with you.
Why do you ask?
I have my reasons, unknown to you.

I don't need to tell you everything,
Some things are best left
Private.

I'll let you know, if and when I'm ready to tell you.
If we get to that stage in our relationship.
It's personal.

Respect my decision.

No.
No sex.
No thank you.
"No" means "no."

Thanks, But No Thanks, I'm Still Looking.

Sometimes it's fun just to look.
Checking it out.
Go for a latte, nothing serious.
Have a conversation.

You can tell a lot about a person over a cup of coffee.
A conversation, getting to know each other.

Know what you're looking for.
Take your time,
Find out what's out there.
Don't get tied down and wish you would have dated more.
Don't give your body to someone you really don't know.

So there's no sex right now.
Save that for someone special.
Or when the time is right.

In the meantime, just keep looking and checking it out.

I Just Want To Cuddle, That's All.

Snuggling and cuddling,
Without the performance and sweat of sex,
To hug and hold,
To spoon,
To talk about the day's events,
To think about tomorrow,
To be tender.

Being sexual doesn't have to mean hot and heavy sex.

Come over here – I've been saving a little spot for you
Right beside me.
Snuggle in; I'll keep you warm.
There's so much comfort in cuddling.

I Don't Want Quantity Sex; I Want Quality.

Some lovers may want lots of sex—
Every day, twice a day.
Others may want attention to detail—
Hot and heavy, slow and easy, quick or fast.

Each of us has a different level of sexual desire,
Different measures of sex appeal
That can change by the hour, the day, the month, the year.

Some may ration their sexy deeds,
Not having it too often.
Less is more,
Quality....
Maybe if I ration it, you'll want me even more.

Is there ever the perfect time for sex?
Most often, not.
Make the time.
Otherwise you'll find you're not getting any.

Whatever your libido,
Find your compatibility and you'll be fortunate.

No sex in the bedroom is a bad thing.

No Sex Until You're Married.

Respect your partner's values.

Sex to those who wait can have many rewards.
Your first partner will be your last.
No worries about sexually transmitted diseases.
It's an adventure and learning together.

Sometimes asking someone to wait for sex until marriage is a difficult choice.
Between the emotions and physical attractions, it can be very difficult to say no.

Go and stand in the freezer or have a cold shower.
Cool off.

Until next time.
Or not until you're married.

You're Not Over Your Last Relationship.

Sometimes we think going into the arms of someone new will take away our hurt.

A failed relationship can be devastating.
When we lose a love, we feel like a failure,
It tests one's confidence.
It may make you feel inadequate,
Or insecure and anxious.
It breaks your heart.
It makes you suspicious.

Know that you're not worthless if you're not dating.

It's only failure if we keep repeating our errors and ways.
Take the time you need and learn from your past mistakes.
Reach out to friends, not lovers.
Take some time for the wounds to heal.
Every time we lose at love, we can become better lovers.

Sometimes you have to be the heart breaker
Versus having your heart broken.
Or, maybe you can learn more from your own broken heart,
Rather than breaking someone's heart.
You can be better than you were before.

Your broken heart does mend.

In awhile, sometimes the only way to cure an old love,
Is to find a new love.

Your Feet Are Cold.

The ultimate sacrifice:
To allow your partner to warm his/her feet against your body,
Or allow their cold hands to seek out your warmth,
Knowing there's nothing worse than ice-cold hands
on your private parts.
And that cold hands and cold feet melt the passion.

But it's been said those with cold hands have a warm heart.

So turn up the heat!

Put your hands under warm water,
Try some socks,
Build a fire,
Soak in a hot bath,
Get under the blankets.

Body heat will increase.
If not, it's hard to make love to an ice-cube.

Your Feet Stink.

How can we be attracted to each other when I'm turned off?
You're not crawling under the covers when you smell.

Turned off by a foul odor,
Smelly feet,
Body odor,
Bad breath,
The passing of gas,
Dirty hands and fingernails,
Uncut toenails,
Poor personal hygiene.

So if you want to get some loving,
Get scrubbed off,
Get between the cracks,
Get squeaky clean.
When you smell clean and fresh,
And have a manicure or pedicure.
Slather on the lotion so your skin is soft.
That's a turn on.

Then you're always welcome
Under the covers with me!

You Won't Say You Love Me.

Some people don't know how to love.
Some are afraid of love.
Some people have a hard time committing.

They don't want to get tied down.
They don't know what love is.
They may have been burned before.
They can't get the words out.

Some can't say the words to express themselves.
Some need commitment before they have sex.

Others can recognize that they don't have to hear the words "I love you."
Deep down,
They know you care deeply.
And that's enough.

If you can't express the words,
Express your feelings through actions.
Show your love.

I Have A Headache.

It's not a migraine,
But enough pain that sex is out of the question.

A salesman once came home after a long trip.
It was late at night.
He went straight to the medicine chest, got some headache pills and opened
his sleeping wife's mouth.

She woke up and asked, "What are you doing?"
"Giving you some Aspirin," he replied.
"I don't have a headache," she said bewildered.
"Oh good – that's the best news I've heard all day!" *

They had some loving!

Don't be the cause of your partner's headaches.
Be sympathetic to your lover's aches and pains.
Exercise, look after your health, and try vitamins
To give you that extra spark of energy.

Lifestyle choices
Can be the cause of some of our physical pains.
Take care of yourself.

* Author unknown

You're Too Shallow For Me.

Some people need to be intellectually challenged,
Inspired.
They need personal growth,
Conversation.
They like to keep up on current affairs,
Engage in politics,
Be with those who are well read.

Shallow and homophobic people turn them off.
Poverty of the mind isn't fulfilling.
Couch potatoes aren't for them.
Or those who wear worn out, shabby shoes.

Other couples are blissfully happy with the one-dimensional,
Being trivial, uninspired, relaxed, and easy going,
Happy with a partner, with the same outlook.

Whatever works for you – whatever is comfortable,
Find the shoe that fits.

You're Having An Affair?!

The trust has been broken.

I can't believe it.
I've shared my life, my love, and my heart.
You're not only hurting me, you're hurting our family.
I feel disbelief.
I was duped.

If you're the unfaithful one,
Recognize that if you do stupid stuff,
You may have to pay the price.

Finding out your partner is unfaithful
Can be a destructive blow.
It erodes your self-esteem.
You feel worthless.
You question, why?
You didn't see it coming.
Why didn't you see the signs?

Now what?
Seek professional counseling.
Talk to friends for support.

It's a choice:
You either walk away,
Or you try to rebuild.
Either way, it won't be an easy journey.
You walk it alone,
Or together.

You're Vulgar And Your Language Makes Me Cringe.

You're crude and profane,
You embarrass me.

Whatever it is, that's bugging you….
It's time to get it off your chest.
Share it with your partner.
It may take some courage, may take some time,
But finally you can say it.

You may be surprised by the reaction.
Your partner may accept your criticism and want to improve,
Or
Just need to realize it or recognize it.
He or she shouldn't ignore it.

So which one are you?

The one who needs to speak up?
Or the one who needs to change?

You're Not Who I Thought You Are.

You're too wild,
Too boisterous,
Too energetic.
You stay out too late.
You party all the time.
You drink too much.
You're too extravagant.
You spend too much money.
You're a tight wad.
You talk too much.
You're too hard on my ears.
You're full of yourself.
You're grouchy or moody.
You're different behind closed doors.
You're not a good fit for me.

No sex for you.

Please don't call me anymore.
Find someone else.

Why waste your time with someone who's unsuitable?

I'm Jealous!

I need to claim you're mine.

Flirting can cause jealousy.
It's a dangerous game.
Flirt with your partner, not someone else.
There are serious risks with a roving eye,
A playful flirt, no matter how innocent and fun,
Can be fatal to a relationship.

Don't try to make someone jealous.

Once your partner feels wary,
They'll keep an eye on you.
Your relationship isn't healthy anymore.
Your partner needs to be able to trust you.

If you're jealous—beware the green-eyed monster.
Jealousy can spoil your relationship.

Jealously can heat things up,
But only if it's in very small degrees.

Otherwise, it's an ingredient that leads the relationship to destruction,
And turns emotions to the highest and sometimes fragile level.

While a little competition can wake up your sleepy partner,
Be careful.

Jealousy can be hurtful.
Jealousy can wound your relationship.

We Argue Too Much.

You're wrong and I'm right.

Yes, we may have a fight
And it turns our emotions into overdrive.
A screaming match isn't cool.

But be careful of the consequences
Of arguing and quarrelling.
Know when you've said enough.
Know when to be silent.

Apologize,
Stand corrected,
Learn to say the words "I'm sorry!"
Care about your partner.
Recognize how they feel.

Don't keep bringing up the details of past arguments.
Don't say "chill" or "relax" when your partner's upset,
It may only flame the fire and heat things up,
But not in a good way.
Take a look in the mirror and maximize your good points
And minimize your bad.

Good relationships can work through differences and aren't afraid of disagreements.
Good relationships understand.
Good relationships put things behind you,
Without bringing up the past, repeatedly.

Make-up sex can be fun,
But abusing make-up sex isn't healthy.

I Cheated On You And I'm Sorry.

The temptations of another's flesh,
Infidelity was chosen.

Things were a bit slow at home.
Life was a bit boring.
So I tried one for old times sake.
Sex with an ex or someone new.

The sex was exciting, hot, passionate and steamy.
It felt dangerous, wicked and wild.
But it cost me.
I'm an emotional wreck.
I feel so guilty with the flashbacks.

What was I thinking?
The affair was a temporary solution for me.
Now I may lose you.
I don't want to move out.
My future could be shattered.
You've lost trust in me.
I wish I could have it all back.
I'd give anything for a do over.

What was I thinking?
Will there be enough forgiveness to get us through this?

We all make mistakes.
Don't make a habit of making this one.
Your partner may forgive you once,
But likely not a second time.

One can choose forgiveness.
Forgive yourself,
And ask for forgiveness.

Can a relationship get through an affair?
Maybe, but it will never be the same.

Sex Isn't Very Good With You.

You lack that tender caring touch.
I need you to be more loving.
We need to try new things.
We're way too routine in our sex life.
I don't want a marriage that's monotonous.
Give me one that's stimulating, not complacent.
I want so much more than just a marriage on paper.

Good sex is experienced and learned.
Bad sexual experiences can stick with you.
Being prudish about sex isn't exciting.

If you don't develop healthy sex habits,
And a good attitude about sex,
You may have problems with your sex life.
But you can always seek help from a therapist.

A vanilla sex life is fine as long as it has flavor,
But too bland with no zest
Won't last.

If sex isn't a priority, maybe it should be.

Along with caring, kindness and warmth.

Your Annoying Habits Are Bugging Me.

Don't floss your teeth in front of me.
Don't spray toothpaste on the mirror.
Don't leave your clothes on the floor.
Don't leave your dirty dishes in the sink.
Don't leave smelly dirty ashtrays filled with butts.
Don't leave your empty beer cans.
Don't' chew with your mouth open.
Don't bite your nails.
Don't leave the toilet seat up (or down)
—depending on your gender.
Don't hog the remote control.
Don't talk on the phone and ignore me.
Don't keep checking your email or Blackberry.
Don't surf the web or play your computer games and forget about me.
Don't play so much poker, I'm lonely.

There are too many negatives here.
Re-think this relationship.

It's never too late to start changing your life—
For the better.

There's Way Too Much Interference In Our Relationship.

A controlling in-law—
Your family is nosy.
Spending too much time at your parent's house
Now that you're married.
Girls' night out,
Guys' night out,
Friends that don't know when to go home.

There's not enough time or space for us;
You and me—a couple?

We need to set ground rules.
And clarify the boundaries.
Let's not let our relationship be controlled by others.

I Don't Feel Close To You Today.

Beware of your partner's moods.
When the day is tough,
When our emotions are low,
Don't say things you can't take back.
Don't be short.
Don't be snippy.
Don't be moody.
Don't be grouchy.
Don't dig yourself a deep hole.
Sooner or later you'll need to crawl out.

There are times in our lives when we may not be cheerful.
But how we deal with it,
And our response
Is significant.

Don't wallow in negativity or despair.
Don't let your moods become routine.

Bad moods are just a passing phase we all go through,
Know when your partner is having a tough time.
Be patient.
Be supportive.
Don't be suffocating.
Breathe.

All partners need space.
They'll come back to you.

I'm Tired Of This Arrangement
And Want Something Permanent.

Sorry, no more dine and dash.
I'm tired of you loving me and leaving me.
We make love and then you make tracks.

Yet, lately you've been leaving your stuff:
A toothbrush,
Personal effects,
A change of clothes,
The extra pair of shoes.
I like that and it makes me smile.

Do you really want to go home and sleep alone?
Do you think it's time for a commitment in this relationship?
Are we thinking the same thing?

Some lovers may have no difficulty with loving and leaving.
Some lovers continue with no strings attached; it's just the sex.
Neither of you are ready for the commitment of a relationship,
But you like the passion.

Whatever works for you,
As long as you're in the same place,
The same headspace.
If not, there are going to be problems.

I Don't Know Your Sexual History.

How much of a player have you been?
What skeletons are in your closet?

Warning! Sex may be extremely dangerous to your health.
Be aware of your partner's health status.
Ask for a blood test.

When in doubt, don't.
Safe sex and a condom are a must.

Don't wake up with a sex hangover
With someone you don't know too well.

I've Lost Someone Very Close To Me.

The loss of someone special is very traumatic:
A parent, a brother, a sister, a relative, a friend, a co-worker
Or a special pet.

Sex is the last thing on your mind
When your heart is a storm of emotion.
There's a void in your heart,
Sadness,
Tears and memories,
What was,
What might have been.

When someone in our circle of love is gone,
Our heart is broken.

It takes time to heal,
Time to grieve.

Give your partner compassion and consolation.
Hold them.
Comfort them in their grief and darkness.

You will see the sunshine again.

Because You Make Me Nervous.

You never know for sure,
First impressions can be wrong.

It's okay to have jitters on your first date,
But once you begin talking, the nervousness should disappear.

Be careful,
If you're not sure, don't date alone.

Most often, men are the stronger sex, physically.
Don't force yourself on someone.
"No" means "no."

Don't try to charm your way to sex
When your partner isn't sure.

Dominating and controlling partners are scary,
And that isn't fun.

Being nervous or anxious is a good reason not to have sex.

I'm Intoxicated And Not Feeling Too Good.

I've tasted the wine and whiskey.

I've tried to drown my sorrows but I keep thinking of you
Time after time.
I know I've made mistakes, way too many mistakes.

After a few hot cups of coffee and a good night's sleep,
I'll come to my senses.

I will always love you.
Give me a second chance.
Love and forgiveness, that's all I ask.

Maybe I'm an alcoholic?
Maybe I have a drug habit?

Alcoholics and substance abusers are a lonely breed.
It's a desperate illness that leaves you with your tears,
Unstable emotions, depression, broken hearts,
And broken dreams.
Alcohol or drugs can only numb your pain, not take it away.
Sooner, if not later,
Your partner will have enough and escape from the relationship.

No one should be a hostage to a partner
With substance abuse.
Seek help for yourself and your partner.

If you're the user, kick the habit.
Seek counseling.
You need help.

You're A Bad Actor.

It's your wild, wicked and dangerous sense of excitement
that intrigues me.

Living on the edge entices me.
I'm curious.

The bad and mischievous one is exciting at first.

But to spend the rest of your life with a bad actor,
a bad boy, a bad girl,
Can lead to a lifetime of heartache and grief.

Don't tie yourself down with a bad one.
You know…. the vibes are dangerous.
Your gut feeling is telling you it's not quite right.
Life will be easier without them.
If you play, you'll pay.

Be ready to pass on these ones.
You'll be glad you did.

You're not interested.

You Make Me Angry.

We all have different levels of tolerance—
We can only take so much.

But when that special someone angers you, all sex is off.
They may know or not know the button,
But it's been pushed.

You squabble, you bicker, you argue, you natter, you whine.
When you're arguing or disagreeing,
It's very important to know when to shut up.
You don't always have to win the argument.
Remember, it's important to know when to be silent
And when enough has been said.

You're not perfect, so don't expect others to be.
We all have flaws and should look in the mirror now and then.
If you don't have anything constructive to say,
Keep it to yourself.

A cold shoulder is hard to break.
Anger frosts communication.

But then there's make-up sex.
Now that's a button to push!
You know now,
The most important button to push is the love button.

You Don't Make Me Happy Anymore.

You shouldn't expect your partner to make you happy.

Happiness and contentment starts within.
You have to love yourself first.
Be fit, be active, do something,
Have your own interests and hobbies,
Be responsible for yourself.
It's maturity.

There's a duty to look after you—both inside and out.
See the glass half full.
Don't fake your relationship.
Be true to yourself and to your partner.
It's how you frame things in your mind.
It's how you react to circumstances.
Don't wait for your partner to make you happy.
Find the contentment within yourself first.
Or your relationship could go South.

Is This As Good As It Gets?

You don't turn me on anymore, so turn me loose.

We live in a throwaway, disposable society;
If something doesn't work, instead of fixing it we discard it.
We get a new one.
We live in an instant society.
I want it now.
Some have lost their patience and aren't willing
to put the time in.

Some always long for the lust and excitement
of a new relationship,
And seek them out continuously.
But there's a cost—
When you move from one relationship to another—
Emotional, physical and financial.

Love is not always like the movies or romance novels.
Passion can wane as time together brings familiarity.
But that's okay, it still works.
Familiarity can be good and comfortable.

Think about this
Before discarding your relationship for a different model;
The next relationship will need repairs, too.

I Feel There's A Ghost In Our Relationship.

You talk about your former lover.
You remember aloud the memories you shared.
Maybe you're comparing your former partner
to your new one.
Or maybe you're just sharing thoughts.
Too much information about past loves and relationships
Can make your partner cringe.

They can take it a bit.
They hope one day your reminiscing words will cease.
If you're truly considerate,
You won't talk about your past relationships.
Your partner really doesn't want to hear about them.

Hopefully, and soon,
You won't have anymore unfinished business
And you'll be truly over them.

Yes, ghosts can appear now and then,
But eventually they must disappear.
Instead, create new memories together,
And there will be ghosts no more.

I Think I'm Infected.

If you even think, you have an infection
Or a sexually transmitted disease (STD)
STOP!
Go to a clinic, see a doctor, seek treatment
Immediately.

No sex for you until you've taken care of your health.

I Don't Want To Fight For You.

Love is not a competition.

You think your partner is worth fighting for?
You think you should throw a punch or pull some hair?

What are you thinking?

Fighting another man or woman for the one you love?

Make love not war.

To fight for someone should mean
Being emotionally supportive,
Understanding,
Persevering,
Communicating,
Using your charm and charisma,
Being kind,
Being attentive,
Building a relationship that doesn't need aggression.
Patching things up if you have a disagreement.

If you feel you have to fight for someone,
Physically fight for him or her,
Be the better person and walk away.

I Have A Broken Heart.

It's bruised, cracked and shattered.

Who doesn't know the story of Romeo and Juliet?
To die for someone?
I don't think so.
It may seem when you have a broken heart,
That it will never heal.
You think you'll never love again.

You will.

Relationships strike to the heart of our emotions.
Broken hearts may bring us to our darkest hour.
We feel lost in a wilderness and can't seem to find our way.
Take time to deal with your hurt, one hour at a time, one day at a time, one month at a time, one year at a time.

Keep telling yourself, "I can get through this,
Every day will be a bit better."

Perhaps you'll never forget your former lover.
Eventually, you will learn to handle the ache, a bit each day.
There'll always be the memories.

As time passes,
We have a tendency only to remember the good times
And forget the bad.
But there's a reason why you're not together.

Beware of the one who bruises and breaks you emotionally.
You deserve better.

You will love again.

I'm Afraid Of You.

Violence has no place in any relationship.

Do you or your partner have tendencies to be violent?
In voice and intent?
Do you or your partner throw things at one another?
Is there physical contact that injures?
Do you or your partner act with any physical and/or emotional violence?
If so, you need help.

Abuse takes many forms:
Name-calling and temper outbursts,
The silent treatment,
Holding back financial support,
Threats, ultimatums,
Violent behavior.

A healthy relationship is what you need and want.
No hitting allowed.

If you're the abuser, keep your hands to yourself.
Be gentle,
Hold your tongue,
Keep your temper in check.
Work on it every day if this is a problem for you.

Seek counseling—that's a brave and important step.
It will lead you away from the hurt and pain.
Call an abuse hotline.
Don't blame yourself for the abuse.

 If all else fails, do your partner a favor—
Move on.
Love and violence just don't mix.
You need to know when to let go,
Walk, no, *run* away.
Stay away.
No going back.

Your Partner Doesn't Want Sex.

If you don't want sex,
It doesn't mean you don't love your partner,
But there's magic missing in your relationship.

If you're not giving it up,
Is your partner supposed to become abstinent?
How long is too long before your next sexual embrace?

It's not a good thing
If you can't remember the last time you shared sex.
It's not a good thing if you don't want to have sex.

We're not all built the same.
Our clocks are different.

But eventually the frustrations of no sex could be problematic.
No one wants to feel neglected.
You can seek counseling or see your doctor,
Or just be satisfied that some of us just aren't interested in sex.
That's okay—
As long as it's okay with your partner.

Otherwise, they may look elsewhere.

You Did Something That Ticked Me Off.

For instance:

Men: You peed all over the toilet seat.
You splattered on the floor.
Clean the toilets and you'll understand.
The modern man sits down at home to pee.
Stop leaving your clothes on the floor.
Please, hang them up.

Women: You keep moving things around.
I can't find my stuff.
You're watching too many of those decorating shows.
You're cleaning out the clutter and I'm missing my possessions.
It's good to be neat,
But before you move things around or throw things away,
Talk to me first.

We should talk about the things that bug us.
They're just little things that can be worked on
To make the relationship better:
With more tolerance,
With more caring,
With more communication.

Talk to each other and get it off your chest.

I'm Watching My Favorite Tv Show.

It's that darn TV excuse again!
Once again, a reason we're not having sex.

If the actors on TV have a better sex life than you have,
There's a problem.

Picking a TV show over your partner,
Can crush and dull the passion.

Timing is important.
Just like scheduling your TV program,
Schedule your time for sex and intimacy.

TV can be your competition in the bedroom.
Reality isn't on the television,
It's right beside you.

Instead, turn the TV off once in a while,
And turn each other on.

You Sent Me On A Guilt Trip.

Mind games,
Pouting,
The silent treatment,
Being miserable,
Raising your voice until you get what you want.

No one wants to feel guilty—
If they don't agree with something,
Or, if they don't give you what you want—
Right now!

Relationships are about talking to each other,
Working things out,
The right time, the right place,
Discussing what's reasonable, realistic and rational.
Play fair.

No one wants a ticket for a guilt trip.
And I'm not making love to you with that pouting face.

I Have A Yeast Infection.

You may not want to hear about it.

Yikes.

It's burning, itchy, wet and uncomfortable.

Best to wait and get treatment before you're intimate.

Take your pills and/or use the cream prescribed.

You'll be better before you know it,

Then you can do the deed.

You're My Worst Nightmare And I Finally Woke Up.

I don't deserve this.
It's not what I've been dreaming of.

Maybe I was first blinded by the sex,
But it's not so great anymore.
The material things you gave me, once delighted me,
But it's just *stuff* now.
The promises of a home filled with possessions,
Isn't fulfilling me.
And really, our home is empty,
And so is my heart.

I want more.
I need more.
I have friends and family who can help me through this.
I'm moving on.

I can't Find My Perfect Match.

You clean up good,
You look your best,
You have charm and personality,

But why are you attracting all the weirdoes?

Or the person is nice, but there's just something missing.
It just doesn't feel right.

Don't despair.
Keep searching.
Be an elephant hunter and search for the best relationship.
Don't settle because you're tired of looking.
Yes, it can be a jungle out there,
But be brave!

It takes time to meet your best match,
Which isn't the same as a perfect match,
Because there can be many well-suited partners out there
For each of us.

You will meet your match.

Then you can light your fire!

You're A Two-timer.

A cheater.
You're juggling relationships.
You can't be exclusive with your partner.

It's a dangerous situation to be in.
You're playing a risky game with too many hearts.

Maybe you can't make the break from one relationship
to another—
You like to live on the edge.

Are you playing a game?
Do you really think you're that incredible?

Maybe you're just a jerk or a user?
Maybe your ego is taking control?
Maybe you don't know a good thing when you have it?
Maybe you're afraid of your relationship?
Maybe you have commitment phobia?

Two timing doesn't work.
Cheating is deception.
You won't be successful.
Put the brakes on.
If you drive two cars at once, you're going to crash.

No one wants seconds.

You've Said You Love Me Too Soon.

New relationships are spontaneous and exciting.
Everything is new—
Affection and admiration,
Feelings and emotions.

Some need more time to grow,
To feel comfortable with the new person in their life.
Take your time.

In a moment of passion, we blurt out the words, "I love you."

Make sure your partner is ready for it.

Intense love and emotions expressed too early
May scare them off.
They can't handle the seriousness.
They can't commit.
They're scared of not being able to play the field anymore.
They don't want someone depending on them too much.
They're scared of losing their independence and freedom.

Expressing love when you know it and feel it is amazing.
Finally....
Finding your mate, your true love.
You feel warm,
Secure,
Confident,
Content,
Fulfilled,
Satisfied.

Don't say "I love you," too soon.
Timing is everything.

You're The Boss And You Call The Shots.

I don't know how it started,
Or how it came to be,
Maybe it's just the natural order,
Where the female sex in a relationship decides,
Sex tonight,
No sex tonight.

The female gets to mind the store.
It stands to reason.
Would you let the fox look after the chicken house?
Or the cat feed the mice?

No.

If you let him have all he wants, he may get tired and lazy—
Take you for granted.

If you ration it out, a little at a time,
He'll keep coming back for more.
You're the boss.
You're in the driver's seat.
You can wear the trousers in your relationship,

But don't be stingy with sex.

You're Not Giving Me My Space.

I feel smothered.
Every move I make,
You have an answer, you have a suggestion.
You watch me all the time.
I feel like I'm in your shadow.

Love is two lives coming together,
Cherishing the closeness,
With respect for your partner's freedom.
Friends and interests outside the relationship are the key.

It's the coming together of two lives,
In a relationship based on trust, sharing and respect.

Being independent is about strength.
Don't be a clinging vine.

Give your partner the room to grow, laugh and love.
Feel good about yourself.
Feel good about each other.

Giving space to your partner
Will be the oxygen your partner needs
To thrive in your relationship.

I'm Moody—Today It's A "No Fly Zone!"

I feel bitchy.
I feel grumpy.
I'm irritable.
I'm menopausing.
No interest in sex.

Moods are like clouds, they move on.
Moods shouldn't be taken out on those we love and care for.
Get your mind off the negative.

Ask your partner, "Do you want to talk about it?"
But don't force the issue.
Be okay with the silence,
Give your partner time to cool off,
When your partner is ready, he (or she) will talk.
Be supportive.
Be sympathetic.
Be patient.

Love is not going to bed angry.
Stay up and talk it out.

Bad moods are a sure bet for no sex.

I'm Seeing Someone Else Right Now.

Be truthful.

Integrity is an esteemed characteristic—
A good golden rule to live by.
Honesty will keep you on track.
Good things will come from the truth.

Don't live your life running and hiding,
Covering one story with another.

Don't keep dark secrets that surprise your partner,
Or haunt you.

Having promiscuous sex isn't healthy.
Don't double dip.

I Feel You're Dumping On Me.

You grumble too much.
You come home and unload all of your problems on me.
You get them off your chest but put them on my shoulders.

Leave your problems at work.
You have to make the transition from work life to home life—
Two different worlds.

Don't make a constant habit of dumping your problems
on your partner.
Recognize that not all problems can be fixed overnight.
They take patience and time.

Yes, we all need to share our problems with someone;
Someone to talk things through,
Or hear a different perspective.
But do it at an appropriate time,
When your partner can give you their time and energy,
To listen to you.

No one wants to hear a complainer,
It's depressing.
And doesn't give good vibes for sex.

You're Too Fussy...

You're too fast.
You're too slow.
You're too hot.
You're too cold.
It didn't last long enough.
You're taking too long.
You didn't warm me up first.
You're too big.
You're too small.
I want everything just right.

If you want perfection—Good Luck!

Find balance.
Accept the blemishes.
We're not all perfect.
Be reasonable and tolerant.

Those unreasonably fussy people,
Get to sleep on the wet spot,
…If there is one.

You're Late Again.

I begin my day with anticipation—
It's going to be a wonderful day.

I put on my best.
I'm lookin' good.
I smell great.
I'm ready.
I can hardly wait to see you.

Your lover is late.
It's a let down,
It spoils the mood.

You know that being late is my pet peeve—
It bugs me.

Sometimes, all you have to do is be on time.
Make your best effort.
Don't take your partner for granted.
Be punctual.
Be considerate.
Know that they can depend on you.

If you're going to be late, make sure you call,
Or come in the door,
Asking for forgiveness,
Or bearing gifts, to make up for lost time.

You Forgot To Bring The Condoms.

If you're too shy or embarrassed to buy condoms,
You're not ready for sex.

Practicing safe sex is serious business.
Plan ahead and take precautions.

Don't play a game of roulette with your sexual health.
No glove,
No love.

Don't take chances with disease or unwanted pregnancy.
It's not worth it.
Seek advice from your doctor.

Have sex another day—when you're prepared.

We Haven't Given It Enough Time.

One partner says:

"That's enough dating; we should have sex."

The other says:

"You can't have sex with me right away,
You have to get to know me first.
Slow down,
Take me out,
Wine me,
Dine me,
The courtship, please!
Kiss me,
Caress me,
Show me your heart,
Show me your patience,
Show me what you're about,
Show me you can wait."

Give the time to know each other.
You'll know when the time is right.

You're Too Controlling.

You're too bossy.

When I think about it, you've tried to control me from day one.

You make the decisions.
You're always in charge.
I feel trapped.
I feel overwhelmed.
I need space.
My spirit is broken.

I see things more clearly now.

I'm not the person for you.
You're not the person for me.

I'm in the driver's seat now.
I'm steering this relationship in the direction
I want it to go.

I've decided I'm moving on.

You Complain Too Much.

You complain about dinner.
You wish I were thinner.
Your eggs are cold.
The bread's too old.
Your back needs rubbing.
The floor needs scrubbing.

The sex is too fast.
You're full of gas.

We're not in sync.
I need a drink.

Will things get better?

It can be so easy to complain.
Take notice of what you say,
You may be the complainer.

Instead, help each other make a better day.
Be part of the solution,
Not the problem.

It's Stormy In Our Relationship.

The winds are blowing ill will between us.
All is not well.
There's pressure in our relationship;
High pressure,
Low pressure,
It's hot,
It's cold....

Let's take a temperature check.

Our life can be better:
To be more tolerant with each other,
To be a better listener.
Give more and want less.
Understanding we're both different,
Appreciating each other more,
Recognizing you make a difference in my life.
Not expecting love to be perfect.

Tensions build—
Give time for emotions to cool down.
Know when you've said enough.
No physical or emotional abuse.
Let your mood be calm and in control.

Storms do pass.
Together, we can weather the storm to sunny days ahead.

We Can't Find The Right Time.

Our jobs,
Our schedules conflict.
I'm an early riser;
You like to sleep late.
I come home,
You're on your way out the door.
Friends,
Family,
Things to do,
We're not spending enough time together.

It feels like we're on a merry-go-round.
We don't know when to get on,
Or get off.
We need give and take.
We need common ground.
Sacrifice a bit for each other.
We need to realize what's most important.
Our fast paced lives?
Or our relationship?

Who wins?
Love and our sex life,
Or the rat race?

You Talk Too Much.

Some of us have a lot to say.
It goes on and on,
Perhaps to the point of verbal diarrhea.
Not pleasant,
Overbearing,
Way too much.

If you think you talk too much, you probably do.

After a while, friends will hide from you,
Make excuses, just to get away.
They don't want to hear that same old story—
Again!

Take a step back,
Take a breath,
Make room for others to talk,
Listen with your two ears,
Think before you speak,
Enjoy the quiet and the silence.

Please, don't talk so much!

I Don't Want To Regret This.

Which is better?
Which is worse?

To regret what we have done?
To regret what we have not done?

We all make mistakes.
Now and then, we choose the wrong path.
To decide on the right path offers great reward.
Taking the wrong path can be difficult,
But if you learn from it,
You can get wisdom and education like no other.
Life's lessons show us the way,
If we keep our eyes, heart and mind open.

A missed opportunity.
A missed love.
A moment that will never come again.
Thinking what might have been.

Take a chance.
Be hopeful
Show courage.
Have strength.

If you've never made a mistake, you've never lived.
Trust your feelings and listen to yourself.
Learn from your experiences.
No regrets.
It's your call!

Which road do you take?

You Owe Me....
I Have A Lot Of Time And Money Invested In You.

If you think your partner is bought and paid for, think again.
Love does not have a price tag.

It would be a worthwhile arrangement to get good value
for your emotional investment,
But there are no guarantees.

Love is a gift of time when we share our love.
Love should be given with no expectations or limitations.

If you expect and demand sex for your investments in the relationship,
You may be in for a hard awakening.

Don't give anything you may want back or trade for sex.

And if the relationship doesn't last,
If the investment goes bad,
It's called "the screwing you get from the screwing you got."

I Lost My Job.

The loss of your job or your partner's job
Can be a shocking experience.
For them,
And for you.

It unsettles your existence.
It shatters your stability.

A job provides you with friendship and financial security that's linked to
your emotional security.
Our work not only provides us with our basic needs of
food and shelter, but also with self-esteem and self-worth.

When our basic needs are threatened,
Who on earth is thinking about sex?

On the other hand, maybe you'll have more time for sex.
Moreover, it's an emotional and physical release.

In the meantime, deal with the stress.
Keep in touch with friends and family—seek their support.
Be positive.
Believe in yourself
Move ahead.
Hug and support each other.
Hang on to the rollercoaster.

You will work again.

There Are A Lot Of Distractions In Life.

Work,
The kids,
Juggling childcare.
Paying the mortgage,
Paying the bills,
Laundry,
Dishes,
Vacuuming,
House repairs,
Family problems,
TV,
School,
Sports,
Pets,
The community,
Out with the boys,
Out with the girls,
Pressures and deadlines....
We multi-task,
Life can be hectic, messy, and a bit crazy.

Your partner should be your main attraction.
Coming together amidst all the activities
Can bring calm to the twists and turns of our lives.

Despite the whirl around you, remember what's important.
Attention to each other is a must.

Someone Threw A Monkey Wrench And It Hit Me.

The monkey wrench is the unexpected.

Those events in your life that seem to pop up from time to time:

- a problem to deal with—personal or work,
- someone from your past coming back into your life,
- a lost loved one,
- a mood that leaves you blue,
- a troubled partner,
- you're getting older,
- illness,
- what's next?

A monkey wrench can try you.
A bump in the road and you didn't see it coming.

When life's mysteries test your love, hang on.
Remember all that you went through.
Remember your first date, your first kiss.
Remember your successes and accomplishments,
How far you've come.
Remember your life's firsts—your child's first words or
first day of school, your first day of driving, and your first love.
Remember who stood with you through love and heartache, good days and
bad days.

We put our relationships through tests.
But if we ask the wrong questions,
We are likely to get the wrong answers.
The best test is the test of time.

When you've had an unpleasant day, you don't feel sexy,
And it doesn't feel like the time for sex,
Remember who gives you support.
Reach over. Embrace.
Try to think positive.

Tomorrow is another day.

We Have Conflict.

Conflict can be exhausting.
How can we deal with it?
We don't always have to agree
But can we find common ground?

Your body language is telling me a lot.
The silent treatment doesn't work.
We need to be able to talk to each other.
We need to be gentle with each other.
We need to be able to tell each other what we really mean—
Plain language,
Honesty.
Not talking in riddles.

Maybe if I wait long enough, you'll understand me.
You need to say what you're thinking.
You can't read my mind.
You can't guess how I'm feeling.
If either of us have something to say, we should say it.
No guessing.
Let's sit down and talk it through.
Communication, please!

Can we compromise?
Can we both give a bit?
Can we agree to disagree?
Can we find a way to make both of us happy?

Conflicts are like bricks.
Anger and resentment need to be pushed away
So they don't weigh on our hearts.
If we don't work through them,
One day the walls will be so high
That we won't see each other anymore.

Can we find a way to work through our differences?

Something Is Missing From Our Relationship.

Our relationship isn't healthy and needs a prescription.
We need to immunize this relationship
Against separation or a divorce.

We're still sleeping in the same bed,
But I feel your detachment,
It's becoming the norm and I don't like it.

Is it because you're preoccupied with your work?
Don't you find me attractive anymore?
Is it something I've done?
Or haven't done?
We can't resolve our problems
Unless we recognize we have them,
Or talk about them, even though that may be difficult.

How much time do we spend on creating our relationship to what we want
it to be?
We need to spend time together.
We need to use kinder words.
We need to treat our partner the same as you would like to be treated.
We need to be appreciative every day.
Good lovers communicate every day.
We need to listen with our hearts.

Are we too busy to connect?
Do we have the commitment to make our relationship better?
The ball's in my court.
The ball's in your court.

I'll wait a while longer, give it some time,
But it takes two of us to make it work.

Let's see if we can find what's missing.

It Feels Like All You Want Is Sex.

Sometimes, that's how women feel.

Be wary of amorous men.

There's something that women should know:
Most men are horny.
They have the insatiable biological desire to have sex.

Young men need only a short time before the next performance.
As the years go by, it takes a bit longer to get that
second wind.
A middle-aged man may be ready to roll by morning.
An older man is glad it works.

No matter what their age—
Their libido, sexual appetite, cravings and desires
Need quenching.

Most men are amorous and want sex—
No matter what their age.

Yes, women too, can be oversexed, fervent lovers,
And use it when they want it.

But normally, it's the male species
That comes first in this category.

You Call Me Names.

You belittle me.
You knock me down a notch.
You make fun of me.
You're on my case.
You pick away,
You chip away at my self-esteem.
My feelings seem to be at the door,
Like a mat on which you wipe your feet.

Does your partner really know what they're doing to you?
Do they care?

Clue them in—
Tell them that that they're hurting you.
Insist on respect.

If you can't resolve things on your own,
Go for counseling, preferably together.

If it doesn't feel good, don't be there.

If no results, show them the door,
Or walk out the door.
You deserve so much more.

I've Got A Lot Of Things To Do.

No time for sex.
I have studying for my education.
My energy is directed to establishing my career.
I have places to go and things to see.
I want to travel.
My family needs me right now.
My friends are more important.
I have no time for you.
I don't want to get tied down.
I'm not ready.

Do the things you want to do before you tie yourself down,
Or settle down.

Enjoy your single life
Before you commit.

Get it out of your system.

You're Saying Bad Things About Me.

I trusted you.

Someone lonely and looking for love and compassion
Can be trashed by cruel gossip.

Partners who brag about their conquests at the expense of someone who
loved and trusted them
Are not worth it.
They're mean and destructive.
Braggarts are inconsiderate losers.

Sex is intimate and should be private.

Learn discretion.
Don't break the trust.
Don't kiss and tell.

You Bug Me.

Yes, you're the bug of the week.
You know all those reasons why I fell in love with you?
Well, now you're really bugging me.

I'm tired of your jokes,
Your inappropriate behavior,
Familiarity,
Snippiness,
Nagging,
Arguing about nothing important;
That's a trap many couples fall into.

Watch yourself.
Part of it is too much work and too much stress,
The every day pressures lower our tolerance levels.

You love your partner,
But you're not in sync.
Sleeping on the couch,
In the doghouse.
Some of you give more respect and courtesy to strangers than family under
your own roof.
Remember that kindness begins at home.
You can have way more fun
Bending over the couch
Than sleeping on the couch.

Don't bug me.

I'm Feeling Neglected.

I'm feeling out of touch.
I'm feeling shortchanged.
I don't feel appreciated.
I'm feeling resentment, frustration and disappointment.
I don't feel loved.

You come home late.
You're hungry and tired.
You don't say much when you eat.
Help around the home is unheard of.

You expect to have sex "on demand."
You wonder what's wrong when you don't get any.
I don't enjoy sex anymore.
I just want it over and done with.
This is not a good situation—
For either of us.

Let's talk to each other.
I want you to know what I'm feeling.
Just because we're not sharing sex,
Doesn't mean the love is all gone.
Pay some attention to the neglect of each other,
And to the relationship.
Do some sex homework and work on solving the problems.
If we can't communicate verbally, let's do it through actions.

Let's create, rekindle and rediscover
The magic between the sheets.

You Won't Take Me Out.

We've been together for some time now.
Our evenings consist of supper, little or no conversation.
TV or newspapers capture your partner's entire attention.
Yoo hoo – there are two of us in the relationship!
It's not enough fun anymore.

It's important to do things together,
Or you'll end up in a rut.
You think it's bad now?
It will only get worse unless you do something.
You'll get cabin fever and want to escape.

Take a walk,
Hold hands,
Take a drive on undiscovered roads,
Enjoy a sunset,
Go for an ice cream,
Take a trip to the library or bookstore,
See a movie,
Visit friends,
Be spontaneous,
Ride the Ferris wheel,
Go for a spin on a motorcycle as you hang on tight
And feel the vibrations,
Play some music and make some noise,
Don't forget the romance,
No matter how long you've been together.

Find some fun outside the home and bring it home.

It will change the energy in your bedroom.

You're Too Wimpy For Me.

"I like it if you like it."
"I'll go where you want to."
"Whatever you say is fine with me."

Make a decision,
Get a backbone,
Find your voice,
Decide what *you* want.

Yes, compromising and getting along
Is important in a relationship,
But don't lose yourself in the process—
Your values, your individuality, your independence.
Take control of what you need and want,
Not someone dictating to you.

The opposite is being the controller,
Everything has to be your way.
You have to be the boss.
In charge and giving the orders.

There's no such thing as a 50/50 relationship.
It's never an equal equation.
Rather, it's about each individual giving or attempting to give 100%
To the partnership.

You Won't Let Me Have The Remote Control.

The silly squabble over which show to watch;
Don't let TV interfere with your sex life.
If it's really a good show, have sex before or after.
Make the time.

Or is holding that remote control
About control in your relationship?

Come to a happy medium,
Compromise or take turns,
Monday is my turn, Tuesday is yours.
Schedule your favorite shows.

Be considerate and share.

If you don't give up control of the TV control box,
You won't get any loving from the love box.

You're Cut Off.

You're in the penalty box.
Go sit in the corner.
You're in the doghouse.

You've been bad;
Came home too late,
Not coming home at all,
Forgot to call,
Drinking too much,
Yelling and using abusive language,
Shopping too much,
Gambling,
Selfish,
Inconsiderate….

If you're just cut off a few days, consider yourself lucky.
A strong relationship can survive some problems,
But when it becomes an ongoing roller coaster ride,
You'll both get tired
And want to get off.
We all have our breaking points when enough is enough.

Cut out the bad stuff,
Focus on being a better person.
Focus on meeting your partner's needs.

Be a better partner, a better spouse.
The game will be more fun,
Without going to the penalty box.

You Haven't Grown Up.

We enjoy our youth—
Lots of energy and crazy ideas.

But youth can be hard on relationships;
Parties, drinking, sports, bars, friends,
late nights and early mornings.

Some never get past the carousing.
They can't say goodbye to the party mode.
The relationship is too crowded,
Because there are too many friends in it.
Responsibility and maturity is lacking.

Most of us grow up.
For some, it can take longer.

Growing up means partying between the two of you,
Changing your old ways.
Two in the relationship,
Two with individuality.
Two coming together
As a couple.

Sharing two lives
Together.

Too Many Lovers.

In our search for love,
We may go round the block too many times.
For some, that's fun.
For others, it's not acceptable.

Some of us can be lucky and find love early.
We find the fit without having to experience too much,
Others are continuously seeking.

We all search for love;
Wanting to be held, understood, comforted and appreciated.
In doing so, some people get the wrong idea.
They take advantage of our vulnerability.

One should be cautious.
Don't give out sex too freely.
Don't be promiscuous.
Don't hate yourself in the morning.
Save sex for someone very special.
Good reputations take time to build.
Don't lose yours by sleeping around.

Not all relationships need to have sex—
At least, not right away.
Be generous in spirit, and not with sex.
Give the relationship time to grow.
The passion will be there
When you're ready.

I Want To Talk First.

Oh no, she wants to have a conversation!
Most women like to talk before sex.
Most women like to talk after sex.
Conversation with sex is important.

Talk about your day, the kids, the neighbors, current events,
dreams and schemes.
Share your thoughts, or talk about your feelings.
Women like that!

Or let her know you don't really feel like talking.
Have your partner cuddle next to you,
Stroke their skin,
Feel the warmth,
And appreciate the silence.
If you do share your feelings,
Make sure they're the right ones!

Dialogue is not always necessary to communicate emotion.
Quiet is sometimes how we are.
Some of us are deep thinkers;
We do more thinking than talking.
In silence there can be bonding.

Enough talking already!
Let's have sex….

And then let's go to sleep.

I'm Tired Of Meeting Losers.

And sometimes I feel like a loser.
Why can't I meet a good one?

Sometimes it may look like all the good ones are married,
Or taken.
Each relationship you have isn't a good fit.
You're frustrated and lonely.
You've been date free for far too long.
You're overeating because it's your way of
dealing with rejection.
You've even taken a short-term vow of celibacy.
Your friends are all getting married.
Your family says you're too picky.
The pressure is on for grandchildren.

In the meantime, keep busy, be active.
Read, volunteer with a charity, take a course or learn a second language,
exercise, work or travel.
Your activities will lead you to new and interesting people.

Be the best you can be.
Make yourself into the person you want to become.
Physically, intellectually and emotionally,
Find your identity.

When you're least expecting it,
Or when you're not looking,
You'll meet that special someone.

Never give up hope.

You've Changed.

When we first meet someone, we're on our best behavior,
Putting our best foot forward,
But there comes a time when we show our true colors.
They come out eventually—
The real you, both inside and out.
You can't keep a secret.
Your character shows itself.

Don't be something you're not.
You should bring out the best in your partner.
Don't be someone who brings out the worst.

There's something to say about the test drive.

It's been said you never know someone
Until you live with them.
Spend some serious time together to appreciate
Or not appreciate them.
Don't be afraid to show the real you.
Come out of your shell.
Bloom like a flower.

Your partner may say you've changed.
Sooner or later the truth comes out.
You may see a different side of each other.
What you see is what you get.
It's an awakening.
It may really mean you're not a good fit for each other.
You've shared time together and made memories.
But then comes the recognition.
It's not a good match
Anymore.
Some relationships last forever, others for a short time.
Time to say good-bye.

I'm Depressed; You Filled Up The Job Jar Again.

It's hard to keep up.
One's home should be a sanctuary, not another workplace.
It should be a hideout from work, a place to unwind and relax.

But there it is—the job jar,
The "honey do" jar,
A constant reminder there's something you haven't done,
Another duty,
Another obligation.
But that's life and reality.
Yes, our home needs love and maintenance.
We can't neglect the details for improvement.

A job jar doesn't have to be a spouse's nightmare;
Instead, put in a few fun tasks, family outings, or opportunities to share good times and laughs.

Don't forget to make a second jar—
The jar of "personal desires."
You and your lover can put in your wishes and desires,
And have fun completing the tasks in your bedroom!

I'm Paranoid.... There's Someone Else....

A quiet phone conversation behind a closed door,
An unexplained meeting or absence,
Too much time on the Internet,
I'm wondering about your emails and want to read them....
A saddened expression,
Your actions make me suspicious.

You're here beside me,
But not with me.

I'm worried about your heart.
I'm worried about my heart.

Is your heart with me or someone else?

Paranoia shouldn't ruin a relationship.
Suspicion can be distressing.
Our minds can play tricks on us—
Building doubt, insecurity and uncertainty.

Are you over reacting?
Are your suspicions valid?
Or a figment of your imagination?

I'm Through Trying; I Give Up.

When only one person is putting all the effort and energy
into a relationship,
Eventually, one realizes you've reached the end of the line.

You can only give so much of yourself and if it's not returned,
Your vessel is empty.

In the beginning, you think you can fix the relationship.
You can make it better,
But soon it becomes tedious.
It's a feeling....
Is your partner taking advantage of you?

Love is a two-way street.
Lots of give and take,
An exchange of kindness and caring.

If you have the energy and can give some more—
Do it.

But if you're at the end of your rope,
Be clear about your needs and expectations.
If no response, move on.

Being lonely in love isn't fulfilling.

We May Be Living Under The Same Roof But Are We Living Separate Lives?

We used to speak the same language of love;
Understanding, communicating, testing each other,
revealing ourselves,
Growing together.

Now there's silence between us,
Unspoken words,
Unshared emotions.

Or the nagging and the bickering,
The routine,
The drudgery—
We've hit a snag.
We're stuck.

It feels like it's you.
Or is it me?
There's no *us* or *we* anymore.

You sit across the table,
You lay beside me,
But there's so much distance between us.
No sex anymore, no passion—
No pizzazz.

Do you remember how it used to be?
Can we build the bridge to bring us together?

I want to experience the love we once shared
Again.

I'd Rather Have Chocolate.

Sex and relationships can certainly be complicated.
You need a partner and
Your emotional, psychological and intellectual needs realized.

Yes, there are expectations,
Needs and strains in the relationship.
There may certainly be obstacles.
With complications along the way.

Yet, sometimes you want an easy solution
To make you feel better.
 It's much easier to get extreme pleasure from chocolate.
There are no strings attached to the sweet.
Yes, it can be sticky too, like a relationship,
But it can be flavorful and give you just as much pleasure.

Chocolate is a quick fix,
Chocolate can affect you –
Both psychologically and physiologically.
It can be a good substitute for sex.

But it may not be in your partner's mind.

You're Reading This Book.

Your partner wonders why.

Is it because you see yourself?
Or is it because you see your partner?
Do you have reasons not to have sex?
Or are they excuses?

Passion, love, trust and romance
Are key ingredients for good sex.
Find balance in your fast-paced life.
Make room for you and your partner.

To have sex?
Or not to have sex?
That's the question.

It's your choice,
And your partner's choice.
Stop talking or thinking about it,
Just do it and enjoy each other!

Time to put the book down.
There are no more reasons,
Or excuses.
Time to reflect and contemplate….
Surprise your partner.
Take him (or her) in your arms.

Find the passion.
Make love.
In the end, it's always love that really matters.

Never lose that loving feeling.

About the Author

Dianne Wyntjes is a romantic at heart. She is also a professional leader from Alberta, Canada who works in labor relations. On a day-to-day basis, Dianne deals with a variety of personalities and characters in her work and personal life.

She has drawn from her life's vast experiences, including conflict resolution and finding solutions, to write this book. She has teamed with her husband Allan to express the female and male perspective of relationships.

In the **101 Reasons To Have Sex & Just As Many Reasons Not To**, Dianne provides uncomplicated and respectful inspiration about sex, relationships and love.

Printed in the United States
65489LVS00002B/346-525